NATURAL ~~~ION
FOR
PERIMENOPAUSE

NATURAL NUTRITION
FOR
PERIMENOPAUSE

WHAT TO EAT TO FEEL GOOD AND STAY SANE

Sally Duffin

The information in this book is not intended or designed to replace medical advice. All foods and supplements are consumed at the reader's own risk. All efforts have been made to ensure the accuracy of the information contained in this book as of the date of publication. The author disclaims liability for any medical outcomes that may result from applying the recommendations given in this book.

© Sally Duffin, 2021

Published by Sally Duffin

All rights reserved. No part of this book may be reproduced, adapted, stored in a retrieval system or transmitted by any means, electronic, mechanical, photocopying, or otherwise without the prior written permission of the author.

The rights of Sally Duffin to be identified as the author of this work have been asserted in accordance with the Copyright, Designs and Patents Act 1988.

A CIP catalogue record for this book is available from the British Library.

ISBN 978-1-9989953-0-1

Book layout and cover design by Clare Brayshaw

Prepared and printed by:

York Publishing Services Ltd
64 Hallfield Road
Layerthorpe
York YO31 7ZQ

Tel: 01904 431213

Website: www.yps-publishing.co.uk

To my clients, from whom I have learnt so much

Contents

	Hello there …	ix
Chapter 1	What the Hell is Perimenopause?	1
Chapter 2	Symptoms	9
Chapter 3	Blood Sugar Balance	15
Chapter 4	Hydration	22
Chapter 5	Toxins & Detoxification	25
Chapter 6	Essential Nutrients & Supplements	32
Chapter 7	Phytoestrogen Foods	41
Chapter 8	The Essential Elements for Every Meal	46
Chapter 9	Sleep	50
Chapter 10	Movement	54
Chapter 11	Emotional Support	57
Chapter 12	Other Therapies & Resources	60
	Recipes	66
	Acknowledgments	69
	References	70
	About the Author	74

Hello there ...

How are you doing?

How are you *really* doing?

Did you sleep well or wake every hour with hot flushes?

Are you getting anxious and forgetful?

Do your jeans feel tighter and tighter?

You are not alone. This is what happens as we head towards menopause – as we become 'menopausers' (new word, hope you like it).

This messy bit (the bit before the actual menopause which is simply the point in time when we haven't had a period for a year) is known as **perimenopause** and can feel like an endurance trial of confusing and random symptoms. From hot flushes, palpitations and anxiety, to weight gain and levels of forgetfulness that cause some menopausers to fear they're developing dementia: perimenopause doesn't mess around.

One minute we're being rational humans, making sensible decisions and knowing what's what. Next minute we're bathed in sweat, gripped with anxiety, and biting back tears – usually at the most inappropriate moment.

As hormonal rollercoasters go, perimenopause is as transformational as puberty, only this time around we've got a heck of a lot more to juggle compared to those heady teenage years of worrying about what to wear on Friday night and whether we'll get served at the pub.

This guidebook is a response to the experiences of hundreds of amazing perimenopausal and menopausal clients with whom I've had the pleasure of working in my nutrition & lifestyle medicine clinic. Many of these clients were already struggling with long-term health conditions (chronic fatigue, fibromyalgia, underactive thyroid, autoimmunity, digestive problems - sometimes all these combined) before finding themselves in the grip of perimenopause and desperate for help.

Their doctors were suggesting HRT (hormone replacement therapy) and/or an attitude of "it's your age, get on with it". Quite how they were meant to get on with 'it' while facing daily, life-altering symptoms is beyond anyone's guess, but there we go. I must add that there are many medical professionals recommending more than just replacement hormones for perimenopause support: counselling for example, or CBT (cognitive behavioural therapy) - and an increasing number recognise the value of nutritional changes and herbal medicine too.

Hormone replacement therapy is a lifesaver for millions of menopausers. If you're one of them, that's great - I'm glad you've found the support you need. If you're thinking of trying it, I urge you to make as many of these nutrition and lifestyle changes as you can first. I think you'll be pleasantly surprised by the difference they make, and if you decide to go ahead with HRT, you will have strong nutritional foundations in place to help your body work with those replacement hormones.

Of course, it's not just women who experience perimenopause and menopause. Many trans people who still have a female reproductive system and aren't taking gender affirming hormones are likely to experience it too, which is why I've opted to use the term 'menopausers' where possible to include all who are experiencing this life-changing process. Because research studies and public health guidance use the gender-specific terms 'women' and 'men', those terms are used in various places too.

The wonderful thing about nutrition and lifestyle medicine is that it's open to all regardless of whether you're taking HRT or not. We all need to eat, drink, breathe, move, and sleep every day, which means we have endless opportunities to positively influence our hormones via food and lifestyle choices.

The recommendations in this guidebook provide specific support to help you adapt and cope with whatever hormonal changes your perimenopause has in store.

I recommend reading the chapters in the order they are written first, then dipping back to the ones you feel are most relevant for you at this time. Take what you need from each one and start making changes at your own pace.

Please don't attempt to implement ALL the changes in one go: there's far too much to think about and it'll probably end in tears. (And there's enough of those already thank you.)

Work within your own capacity for change.

If you're super busy and maxed out by life, start with one food swap and one lifestyle change. Stick with those for a week or two before adding in another couple of changes. If you can handle more than this, try two or three food changes and two lifestyle suggestions and see how you get on for a week or so before adding any more into the mix.

Going step-by-step gives the new habits and behaviours time to take root in your daily and weekly routines. This may feel like slow progress, but slow progress is better than no progress, and far better than taking on more than you can handle and ending up weeping in a cupboard.

If possible, find a perimenopausal friend or friends – or anyone who knows what it's like to be at the mercy of hormones – and work your way through the book together. Celebrate each milestone no matter how small – only three hot flushes last night, wahoo! – and keep each other on track when life feels overwhelming. Maintaining diet and lifestyle changes can be hard work and there's a high chance of relapse unless you exercise those self-discipline muscles or have a good friend nudging you back on track – preferably both.

Tell your friends and family about what you're experiencing too. A report from the British Medical Association [1] revealed a strong pattern of highly experienced female GPs leaving their jobs because they were struggling to cope with menopause symptoms with no support from management or peers. Many of them felt afraid to seek help in their male-dominated work environments for fear of being seen as unable to cope. This is a pattern being repeated across countless sectors in society, and it reinforces the untruth that women of a certain age just aren't up to the job.

The more open conversations we can have about perimenopause and menopause, the faster we will see a tidal change in society's attitudes towards it. This is finally happening with mental health, and we need it to happen for perimenopause and menopause too.

These conversations need to involve everyone: from partners, children and close friends to employers and colleagues. The only way we can dispel the many myths around menopause is to value ourselves, prioritise our own needs, and speak out about our experiences.

I hope this book helps you to understand what's happening in your body and how to face these changes head on. I want you to feel **empowered** and **equipped**: able to nourish yourself through perimenopause, menopause, and beyond.

Whatever symptoms you are dealing with, know this: your body is always trying to get back in balance. These symptoms are a sign that your body is trying to find its new 'normal' in an ever-changing environment of hormone havoc. It will get there, and you can help it by giving it the food, nutrients, movement, and rest it needs.

Ready?

Let's begin.

CHAPTER 1

What the Hell is Perimenopause?

We're all clear about what menopause is (the end of periods - yay!), but what's perimenopause?

Well, menopause doesn't just happen overnight. There's a build-up beforehand and a finding-your-feet bit afterwards. Actual menopause is the point at which you haven't had a period for at least 12 months - so in truth, this bit could happen overnight.

This is the normal pattern of hormones over the course of a monthly menstrual cycle, starting on day 1 of the period:

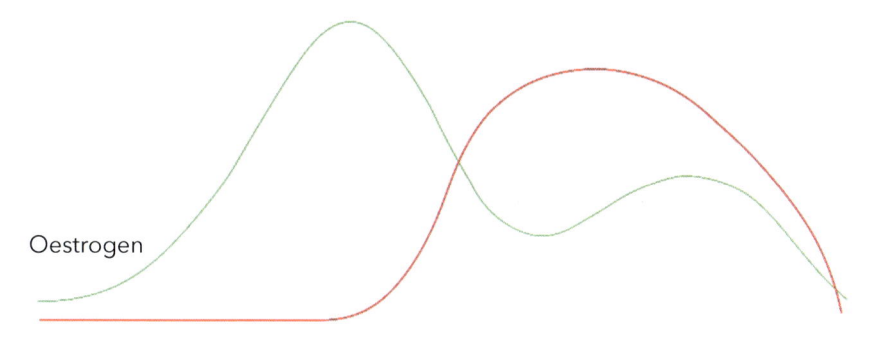

Oestrogen

Progesterone

The oestrogen levels gradually build up in the first half of the cycle (the follicular phase), peaking at ovulation which is round about day 14 on a 28-day cycle. They drop down in the second half, rise again slightly and then tail off as the next period starts. Progesterone on the other hand, doesn't kick into action until the second half of the cycle. After ovulation it rises sharply, peaks, and then tails off just before the next period.

Alongside oestrogen and progesterone, we also have cortisol and the thyroid hormones influencing our energy levels, weight balance, mental well-being, and resilience to stress. Each one has a knock-on effect on the others which is why this book includes guidance on managing stress (hint: if you're dealing with menopausal weight gain, stress management is vital because cortisol encourages weight to sit around your belly) and how to investigate thyroid hormone levels.

Moving to a different groove

By the time we reach our mid-30s/early-40s, the rhythms of our monthly hormonal groove are starting to shift. Rather than dancing harmoniously every month, oestrogen and progesterone start to break out some expressive free-form moves. Things get wild. Perimenopause has arrived on the dance floor.

Perimenopause

Perimenopause is the bit that causes all the bother. This is the transition phase from fertile years to menopause, bringing hot sweats, mood swings, exhaustion, forgetfulness, breast pain, erratic periods, and all manner of havoc (see Chapter 2). It can last for anything from a few months to several years – even a decade – before actual menopause is confirmed.

Perimenopause can begin at any point between the mid-30s and late-40s. Early signs of the new dance moves include changes to mood patterns and anxiety, changes in premenstrual symptoms, and fluctuations in period frequency and flow.

You may not easily detect these signs if you have pregnancies during this time or use hormonal contraceptives that artificially regulate or suppress your hormones.

During perimenopause we are no longer ovulating every month, which means we no longer produce the same amounts of progesterone. This leads to a temporary state of **oestrogen dominance**. This might sound odd given that oestrogen levels are dropping too, but it's all relative.

Progesterone and oestrogen work in relative balance to one another. Once progesterone drops, there's nothing to counterbalance oestrogen. So, during cycles where there's no ovulation, there are relatively higher levels of oestrogen.

As we move through perimenopause, oestrogen gradually starts to decline too, and eventually plateaus out at a much lower level. This chaotic dancing pattern of oestrogen and progesterone is what gives us perimenopausal symptoms.

Menopause

The Main Event. Average age: 52. Most menopausers reach this point between the ages of 45-55, and you may find you follow a similar pattern to your mum or sisters.

Hormone levels are settling down, you haven't had a period – even a light bleed – for well over a year. You're all done! Gift any leftover tampons and sanitary pads to younger friends and embrace this next chapter. No need to plan your life/sex life/wardrobe around premenstrual bloating and unexpected visits from Aunt Flo.

You'll still be producing small amounts of oestrogen from your adrenal glands and fat cells, but these are nowhere near the amounts that were produced by your active ovaries.

Before we get too carried away, there is a bit of a dampener here: some menopausers do still experience symptoms such as hot flushes and mood swings for several years after their last period. Here's hoping you're not one of them.

Post-menopause

Life after menopause! During this stage it's still important to focus on staying active, eating well, and supporting emotional well-being because we can no longer rely on the extra protection oestrogen previously provided. We have oestrogen receptors throughout our bodies, they're on bones, in the brain, digestive tract, vagina, skin, heart, lungs, bladder, blood vessels – everywhere! This is why we can experience such a vast array of perimenopausal symptoms, and why so many areas of our health change post-menopause.

Heart disease – more of a problem than you might think

Heart disease is a major concern post-menopause. Oestrogen helps keep our blood vessels supple and responsive to changes in blood pressure, helps reduce inflammation and plaque build-up in arteries [2], and plays a key role in maintaining healthy cholesterol levels. Once our oestrogen levels drop, we no longer have this level of protection, and our risk of developing high blood pressure and heart disease increases. In fact, the rate of high blood pressure (hypertension) in post-menopausal women is more than twice that in pre-menopausal women [3]. Add in other factors such as smoking, stress, lack of exercise, and diabetes, and we start to see why **heart disease kills more women than breast cancer does.**

On top of the physical changes that make heart disease such a significant issue for menopausers sits the spectre of gender and healthcare inequality. Many gender inequalities exist in healthcare including:

- Difficulties for women in getting their symptoms taken seriously and appropriately managed by health professionals

- Women being more likely than men to be told their symptoms are psychosomatic ("all in the mind")

- Lack of inclusion of women in biomedical research trials which results in medication dosages and effects being suitable for men, but not women

- Lack of support and understanding of perimenopause and menopause symptoms.

Heart disease is a good example of these inequalities at play. There's a strong misperception that heart disease and heart attacks predominantly affect men. This is true pre-menopause, but we soon start to catch up in the ratings post-menopause. Another misperception is that men and women have similar cardiac symptoms. There is some crossover here, but women often experience quite different signs of cardiac problems and may not recognise them as easily.

Jessica Powell, Senior Lecturer in Nursing (Critical Care and Cardiology) at University of York explains in more depth:

"Women frequently experience different heart attack symptoms from men. We tend to think of a heart attack causing crushing central chest pain and pins and needles extending down the left arm. These are the symptoms we are warned about, most often, by public health campaigns. Evidence suggests however that while these symptoms are commonly seen in men, women often experience heart attacks differently. Cardiac symptoms for women can include:

- Discomfort rather than pain (referred to as 'non pain' in medical literature)

- Back pain/discomfort

- Jaw pain/discomfort

- Upper epigastric discomfort (the epigastric region is the upper abdomen, between the bottom of your ribs and your tummy button)

- Nausea and vomiting.

If a woman does seek help for these symptoms, neither she nor the healthcare professional might recognise them as being signs of a heart attack. If they are not recognised and diagnosed, the correct tests won't be carried out.

Diagnosis usually includes one or more ECG tracings and a detailed history from the patient. If neither the patient nor the healthcare professional recognise the symptoms as suspicious, it is quite possible that there will be delays in seeking medical care or that they miss out on life saving – or heart muscle saving – treatments.

Gender-based inequalities also exist in relation to aggressive treatment of their disease and access to cardiac rehabilitation, post event. As such, the implications for women in terms of both mortality and morbidity are significant." [4]

Research by the British Heart Foundation has found that because of gender inequalities, women are about half as likely as men to receive recommended heart attack treatments. Because of this, more than 8000 women have died unnecessarily from heart attacks in England and Wales over the past decade [5].

Looking after our hearts with the right foods and fluids (see Chapter 4 - Hydration and Chapter 6 - Essential Nutrients & Supplements), exercise & relaxation, and stress management is imperative, both before menopause and for the rest of our lives afterwards. If there is any history of heart disease or heart attack in your family, or you are concerned by the symptoms listed above, seek medical help immediately. It might be something or it might be nothing; either way, it's far better to be safe than sorry.

Bone strength

Oestrogen and testosterone (which also drops during menopause) both influence bone-building cells called osteoblasts. Healthy bones are maintained by two types of bone cell: bone builders (osteoblasts) and bone recyclers (osteoclasts). These cells work in harmony to build new bone and breakdown old bone. When bone building doesn't keep up with the rate of bone breakdown, bones gradually become weaker and more porous, leading to the development of osteoporosis - quite literally 'porous bone'.

Post-menopause, we have a much greater risk of bone fractures than men of the same age simply because we haven't got as much oestrogen and testosterone stimulating our bone-building cells any more. Exercise and good nutrition are vital here: the right foods can supply bone-building nutrients, while exercise helps to stimulate those osteoblasts - more on this in Chapter 10 - Movement.

Should I see my GP about perimenopause?

There isn't a clear-cut answer to this question. If you are concerned about osteoporosis, hormonal cancers, unexplained pain or bleeding, palpitations, or any perimenopausal or menopausal symptom then yes, see your GP immediately.

Doctors can test hormone levels but do bear in mind that these results can only show what your levels were at the point the test was taken. The whole point of menopause is that it causes hormone fluctuations, which means snapshot blood tests can be unreliable.

If you feel comfortable riding the wave of perimenopause yourself and don't want HRT then no, there isn't a requirement to see your GP.

Can I take HRT and still follow the tips in this book?

Absolutely! All the nutrition and lifestyle tips in this book are perfectly suitable to follow alongside HRT unless otherwise stated.

Menopause & other health issues

Hormonal changes around perimenopause and menopause can impact other health concerns and conditions. For example, thyroid problems, mental health, digestive issues, and autoimmune conditions (e.g., rheumatoid arthritis and psoriasis) can be affected by perimenopause. Some menopausers find these issues improve, whilst for others the symptoms get worse.

Symptoms of an **underactive thyroid** (hypothyroidism) are often mistakenly diagnosed as perimenopausal symptoms and subsequently not investigated properly.

Signs that your thyroid may not be functioning as well as it should include weight gain, elevated cholesterol, joint pain and stiffness, difficulty losing weight, dry skin, dry hair, poor memory, brain fog, extremely low energy not refreshed by sleep, constipation, breathlessness, and iron-deficiency anaemia.

A lot of these symptoms match those of perimenopause so you can see where the confusion occurs. If you are concerned about thyroid health, ask your GP for blood test investigations. The tests may cover:

- **T4** (both free and total): one of the main thyroid hormones. It is converted in the liver, muscles, heart, and gut to T3, a much more biologically active hormone. T4 production and conversion depend on adequate levels of iron, selenium, and zinc so if you're low in any of these nutrients, your thyroid function may be affected.

- **T3** (both free and total): the more active thyroid hormone. The conversion of T4 to T3 can be disrupted by elevated levels of cortisol (usually caused by chronic stress) and inflammation. Checking T3 levels isn't standard practice in the NHS so you may need a private test for this.

- **TSH**: Thyroid Stimulating Hormone; the chemical messenger sent from your brain to your thyroid telling it to produce hormones.

Elevated TSH levels are showing that your brain is shouting at your thyroid to hurry up and make more hormones. This is one of the first signs of an underactive thyroid gland.

- **Thyroid autoantibodies**: if hypothyroidism (high TSH and low T4) is suspected, it's important to test for autoantibodies to discover whether the immune system is involved. **Hashimoto's Disease** is caused by the immune system mistakenly attacking the thyroid, destroying cells, and causing symptoms of hypothyroidism. If this is the case, you don't just have an underactive thyroid, you have an autoimmune condition affecting your thyroid – this is a completely different situation that calls for an holistic approach to both immune *and* thyroid support.

- **Iron**: both ferritin (the storage form of iron, found in your liver) and haemoglobin (your circulating iron levels) need to be checked.

- **Vitamin B12** – hypothyroidism can affect B12 absorption. Vegans and those taking heartburn medications (Omeprazole, Zantac, Lansoprazole, Nexium) need to be mindful about B12 and may need supplementation.

- **Vitamin D** – low levels of vitamin D are often seen in patients with underactive thyroid and those with overactive thyroid. We know that vitamin D is needed for immune health, but it's not clear whether insufficient vitamin D causes thyroid problems directly, or whether low levels of vitamin D impair immune function and contribute to autoimmune problems affecting the thyroid. Low levels of vitamin D are also a cause of joint pain and inflammation, common symptoms of underactive thyroid. Either way, many people in the UK are deficient in this nutrient, especially people with darker skins and those who are housebound, so it's worth getting tested. It's advisable for all adults and children to take vitamin D supplements between October and April because the winter sunlight isn't strong enough to stimulate vitamin D production in our skin.

If you are already managing an underactive thyroid, be aware that your medication requirements may change as you go through perimenopause and menopause. Those annual thyroid check-ups are important as you may need to tweak your dosages.

CHAPTER 2

Symptoms

Perimenopausal symptoms. Where to begin? They are as diverse and wide ranging as we are.

This is a comprehensive, but by no means complete list of the joyful symptoms perimenopause can bring. **If you are concerned about any of the symptoms in this list, see your GP straight away**. Far better to have something investigated and gain peace of mind than to worry unnecessarily. There is quite a crossover between symptoms of perimenopause and other health conditions so if you have any doubts, get checked out.

- Hot flushes and sweats
- Joint pain and stiffness
- Heavier periods
- Lighter periods
- Longer periods
- Shorter periods
- Breast pain
- Palpitations
- Mood swings and irritability
- Feeling emotionally flat
- Anxiety – often accompanied by feelings of jitteriness

Depression

Poor memory and concentration

Headache & migraine

Insomnia

Dizziness

Nausea

Fatigue

Loss of libido

Vaginal dryness and soreness

Bladder weakness and urinary incontinence

Weight gain – particularly around the belly

Dry/greasy/spotty skin

Weak brittle nails and hair

I think we need to lie down after all that.

The reason why perimenopausal symptoms are so vast and varied is down to the fact that oestrogen influences so many organs and systems in the body. Female hormone expert Dr Felice Gersh [6] describes oestrogen as the 'glue' that binds our reproductive and metabolic systems together, co-ordinating their responses and influencing everything from weight gain and energy production, to bladder function and cholesterol balance.

And oestrogen is more than just a hormone; it also has powerful antioxidant, anti-ageing, and anti-inflammatory actions. Once our levels start to fluctuate, we lose the stability and protection oestrogen brings – and that's when the chaos begins.

Oestrogen & Your Brain

In her excellent TED talk, neuroscientist Lisa Mosconi [7] talks about many perimenopausal symptoms originating in the brain. Our brain and ovaries are communicating constantly as part of what's called the neuroendocrine system. Once oestrogen levels start to fluctuate, the brain receives lower amounts of oestrogen, which in turn causes different symptoms depending on which areas of the brain are affected.

So, when there isn't enough oestrogen to activate all the oestrogen receptors in the part of the brain that regulates body temperature - the hypothalamus - we experience hot sweats and flushes. If there's not enough for the hippocampus, we get memory problems and forgetfulness. Oestrogen fluctuations affecting the amygdala give us mood swings and anxiety.

These symptoms - and all the others in the list - may come and go in a seemingly random way and may change as you move through perimenopause. This is quite normal, it's all down to those dancing hormones.

The important thing to remember is you are not going mad. Yes, your brain is being affected by perimenopause, and yes it may even feel like you no longer have a functioning brain some days, just a head filled with wool, but rest assured you do and it's hard at work adjusting to the new state of play.

The Perimenopausal Vagina

Of all the symptoms listed above, the vaginal symptoms are easily the least talked about. The perimenopausal vagina remains a hidden mystery to many - doctors included. It's as if there's an extra layer of embarrassment here that hot flushes and forgetfulness don't carry. And let's face it, many of us have grown up with minimal discussion (if any) of things like vaginal discharge and vaginal infections, so it's a stretch to think we will be comfortable asking for help with a sore, painful vagina, especially if the GP isn't comfortable chatting about it either.

But the problem is the longer we remain silent the longer it will be before research and resources are directed towards these issues. If you don't feel comfortable talking to your GP, ask to see the practice nurse instead; the likelihood is they will be used to talking about and looking at vaginas. Confiding in friends is important too. You never know who else is struggling but too afraid to speak up, or who else has the same problem and has already discovered a great solution.

Of course, the first part to dealing with any problem is understanding what's happening, so let's delve into the perimenopausal vagina (no, wait, that doesn't sound right at all!) and find out what's going on …

Membranes & Microbes

There are billions of microbes living in your digestive system and vagina, collectively and respectively known as the gut microbiota and the vaginal microbiota. There's a delicate balance of bacteria and yeasts thriving down there, which can be upset by stress, antibiotics, hormone fluctuations, and gut problems. Unfriendly bugs can easily migrate from the gut to the vagina and urinary tract thanks to the anatomical positioning of the anus (always remember to wipe front to back, never the other way!).

There are several residential vaginal bacteria species, one of the main ones being *Lactobacillus* which naturally produce lactic acid. Lactic acid maintains an acidic pH level in the vagina and keeps other microbes in check. Our dancing hormones can affect the balance of vaginal bacteria, which in turn affects acidity levels. Changes to this acid-alkaline balance allows other microbes to thrive, causing problems such as thrush and urinary tract infections.

We normally experience a few changes in the acid-alkaline balance during a menstrual cycle (period flow causes it to go more alkaline) which is why many women experience cystitis and thrush during their period. During perimenopause, this change can last longer, and cause more persistent problems.

Alongside microbial activity, there are a few structural alterations happening to the perimenopausal vagina, labia, and vulva. Essentially, things are shrinking and becoming more fragile:

- The vagina itself gets shorter and narrower
- The lining of the vagina loses elasticity and can become hypersensitive to touch and pain

- Fewer secretions and discharge are produced, leading to vaginal dryness

- The vaginal lining gets thinner and more prone to inflammation and small tears

- The labia and vulva lose plumpness

- The labia and clitoral hood can shrink

- And finally, the pelvic floor loses strength which can lead to vaginal and/or bladder prolapse.

There's an awful lot happening down there that we need to be talking about! These changes are minor for some menopausers but debilitating for others. Severe bouts of dryness and inflammation can make it difficult to wear underwear or any form of trousers; it can be horrendously painful to exercise, and impossible to enjoy sex. Smear tests are never pleasant at the best of times, but with vaginal dryness and fragility they become excruciating. Our vaginal symptoms deserve as much focus and attention as all the other perimenopause symptoms, and there are many ways to help ease the discomfort.

Looking after your vagina

To help manage pain, inflammation, and dryness, the guidance in the following chapters will be helpful:

- Chapter 4 – Hydration: managing any kind of inflammation and soreness requires plenty of good hydration.

- The section on comfortable bowel movements in Chapter 5 – Toxins & Detoxification. Supporting the gut microbiota has a positive ripple effect on the microbes in your vagina and urinary tract.

- Chapter 6 – the section on hair, skin, and nail health in the Essential Nutrients chart, plus information on red clover and omega-7 in the supplements chart.

- Chapter 7 – Phytoestrogen foods.

- Chapter 12 has information on vaginal lubricants, and pelvic floor support.

Alongside these tips, consider using fragrance-free, chemical-free bodywash (or even just plain warm water) to reduce irritation, and opt for organic cotton sanitary pads or washable organic cotton fabric sanitary pads for comfort during periods.

Some vaginal lubricants are available on prescription, so do ask your GP or practice nurse. If you need to go for a smear test, ask the nurse to use the smallest speculum possible, and add extra lubricant.

CHAPTER 3

Blood Sugar Balance

As you've probably grasped by now, there's some hot dance moves happening between hormones every day during perimenopause. And if one dancer is out of step, it causes a knock-on effect on the rest of the dance floor.

It's easy to add to the dance floor chaos by skipping meals, not eating enough, relying on sugary foods and caffeine to get through the day, and using alcohol to wind down at night. We're not designed to handle uppers and downers all the time; humans function best on steady fuel and natural daily rhythms.

Relying on refined sugary foods and stimulants causes spikes of insulin - our blood sugar-balancing hormone - and cortisol, one of our main stress hormones. In turn, these two have knock-on effects on oestrogen and thyroid hormones. Fluctuating blood sugar levels affect our dancing hormones and can trigger many perimenopausal symptoms, including hot flushes, anxiety, weight gain, and forgetfulness.

Let's start with carbohydrates and their effects on blood sugar levels. All types of carbohydrate (bread, potatoes, pasta, rice, etc.) are eventually broken down into simple sugar molecules. These sugars flow through the bloodstream and are ushered into cells by the hormone insulin. Once inside cells, the sugars are used to produce energy (proteins and fats are also used in energy pathways but we're just focusing on carbs here).

If we eat three meals a day composed of protein, fat, and complex carbohydrates (wholefood carbs rather than processed refined foodstuffs), a normal pattern of blood sugar levels looks something like this:

It's a gentle pattern with smooth undulations, and the normal rise-and-fall of blood sugars linked to hunger, eating, and the slow release of sugars from complex carbs.

If we ping-pong through the day on caffeine and refined sugary foods like white bread, cakes, biscuits, sweets, and fruit juices, the pattern looks more like this:

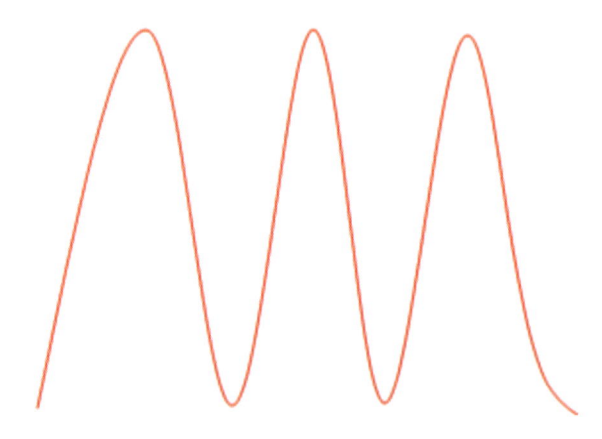

Sharp peaks and deep troughs triggered by rushes of sugar and overworked insulin.

These peaks and troughs can trigger all manner of symptoms including headaches, hot flushes, jittery shakes, irritability, mood swings, and nausea.

As if this wasn't enough, these ups and downs can also encourage **belly fat**.

Every time blood sugar drops too low, we put ourselves into a state of stress, forcing the body to release cortisol, our stress management hormone. Cortisol enables us to tap into stores of glucose in the liver and muscles and bring our blood sugar levels back up a bit. This process is a quick short-term way of managing the occasional bout of low blood sugar. Long term though, ongoing stimulation of cortisol encourages weight gain around the belly area. This is a protective mechanism: if we can't rely on regular fuel, we need to store some energy supplies (i.e., fat) near the important organs. So, the key point to remember here is that **erratic blood sugar levels = stress = belly fat.**

Another problem with running on blood sugar highs and lows is that, eventually, cells start to ignore insulin and it can no longer transport sugar into the cells quite so efficiently. Once this happens, you're on the path to **insulin resistance** and the early stages of Type II diabetes. Oestrogen affords us some protection from insulin resistance because of the way it supports the activity of glucose transporters in cell membranes (these are carriers that aid the movement of glucose into cells), but once oestrogen levels start to decline, we are at much greater risk of developing insulin resistance. Unfortunately, both belly fat and insulin resistance contribute towards general inflammation and the risk of developing cardiovascular disease, so it really is vital to get a handle on blood sugar balance now to help prevent problems developing later.

How to support blood sugar balance

- Eat a balanced breakfast within two hours of waking.

- Avoid (or minimise as much as possible) refined processed carbohydrates: white bread, white pasta, cakes, biscuits, sweets, added sugar, fruit juices.

- Sit down to eat, take three slow deep breaths before your first mouthful, and focus on what you are eating. Chew each mouthful thoroughly until it's mushy and soft. By **eating mindfully**, you are allowing your body to focus on digestion and the signals coming from your stomach that tell your brain when you're full. Eating on the run overrides these signals, leading to indigestion, bloating, wind, and overeating.

- Eat sustaining meals with a gap of roughly four hours in between each one.

- **Avoid snacking** unless there is a gap of more than 4-5 hours between meals. Snacking and grazing triggers constant insulin release and can interfere with digestion (see Chapter 5 for more on this).

- Eat all your meals within a 12-hour time window (e.g., breakfast at 7.30am, last meal of the day finished by 7.30pm) to give your body a 12-hour **overnight fast**. Short fasts like this have been shown to support metabolic function and weight balance and aid digestion (see Chapter 5).

- If you're having **alcohol** (and remember, it's a common trigger for hot flushes), drink it with a meal to help slow down the release of sugars into your system.

- At each meal, think about **portion sizes** on your plate: there's more detailed information and a diagram about this in Chapter 8 – The Essential Elements in Every Meal.

  The general guidelines are:

  - Cover half of your plate with brightly coloured vegetables and salad leaves

  - Cover a quarter with good quality protein sources – eggs, meat, fish, nuts, seeds, pulses, legumes

  - And the last quarter is for complex carbohydrates in the form of root veggies and wholegrains

  - Include healthy fats too:
    - drizzle extra virgin olive oil over cooked veggies and salads
    - Make dressings from flax oil, apple cider vinegar and lemon juice
    - Cook using coconut oil, ghee, or organic free-range butter

- **Fruit** is delicious and healthy, but best limited to three servings per day maximum. It is easy to fill up on fruit at the expense of eating vegetables which are way more nutrient dense.

- If you need **a snack** opt for something unprocessed that combines protein with slow-releasing sugars:

  - Hummus & oatcakes
  - Vegetable crudités & avocado dip

- Hardboiled egg with tomato salsa dip
- Handful of nuts & seeds and a serving of fresh fruit
- Small pot of full-fat live yoghurt (or dairy-free equivalent) with berries
- Handful of homemade trail mix: shredded coconut, almonds, cashews, raisins, dried apricot, and pumpkin seeds
- Homemade smoothie: blend together one small banana, one dessertspoon of nut butter, a generous handful of baby spinach and 250ml of milk or dairy-free milk.

A quick note about dairy

If you are eating dairy products like milk, cheese, cream, yoghurt, and butter, they count towards the protein sources. However, dairy products are all slightly different in terms of nutritional value and the effect they have in the body once digested. Live yoghurt, for example, contains beneficial bacteria that support digestion and immunity and it is higher in protein and lower in lactose (milk sugar) compared to regular milk.

Cow's milk (along with wheat, egg, and soy) is a common allergen and food intolerance/sensitivity. There's a distinct and vital difference between an allergy and an intolerance or sensitivity: an allergy means the immune system is responding aggressively to a protein or proteins in a certain food and the reaction can be life-threatening. Total avoidance of the food trigger is the only safe course of action. An intolerance or sensitivity can cause uncomfortable and distressing symptoms, but these are not life-threatening and the reaction doesn't always involve the immune system. Lactose intolerance, for example, is caused by a lack of lactase, the digestive enzyme that breaks down lactose in the small intestine. When there isn't enough lactase available, the milk sugar carries on through the gut, causing wind, cramps, bloating and diarrhoea.

Interestingly, there are many anecdotal reports from women who say reducing and even avoiding dairy during perimenopause eased their hot flushes. Why this is we're not entirely certain, though a possible theory is that a low-grade inflammatory response to certain proteins in cow's milk may trigger histamine release which in turn can trigger flushing.

If you suspect cow's milk may be causing problems, try a simple elimination test. Avoid all cow's milk products (milk, cream, yoghurt, butter, ice cream, whey, cheese) for at least a month and keep a note of any changes to your symptoms.

If things improve, try slowly reintroducing the products and again keep a note of any changes to your symptoms. If the symptoms come back, you have your answer!

Cheese, yoghurt, and other dairy products can be significant dietary sources of calcium. However they are not the only sources. During the elimination test, experiment with including other sources of calcium in your diet (see Chapter 6 – Essential Nutrients) and if you decide to be dairy-free long term, consider working with a registered nutrition practitioner who can give you personalised nutrition recommendations that meet your needs. See Chapter 12 for how to find a nutrition practitioner.

A quick note about fat

For the past 30+ years we have been indoctrinated into thinking all fats are bad and must be minimised, especially when trying to lose weight. Thankfully, these misleading ideas have now been discredited, but public opinion takes a long time to change.

Yes, fats are high in calories: 9cal per gram in comparison with 4cal per gram for both protein and carbohydrate. But food is way more than just calories, food is information for our cells. We need fats for energy, brain function, skin health, mood balance, and hormone production. Every single cell in our bodies is surrounded by an outer layer made up of fats: when this membrane is attacked by inflammation or infection, cells simply cannot work properly. End of.

Low-fat processed foods are deeply problematic to health. Fat, sugar, and salt are the magical trio of ingredients in processed foods, delicately balanced within each product to optimise taste and texture. When fat is removed, it is replaced by either more sugar or more salt to maintain this balance.

By eating processed low-fat foods for the past few decades, we have created another problem for ourselves: high-sugar diets. And what is excess sugar stored as? Fat.

Healthy fats such as those found in cold-pressed seed oils, oily fish, nuts, seeds, coconut oil, organic butter, and ghee are a vital part of a balanced way of eating. The ones to avoid as much as possible are trans-fats, margarines, and deep-fried foods – especially if they've been deep fried in a polyunsaturated seed oil like sunflower oil. Polyunsaturated oils are always liquids and are easily damaged by high temperatures. This is why saturated fats, those that are solid at room temperature like butter, ghee, and coconut oil, are preferable for baking and roasting. Keep the polyunsaturated sunflower, rapeseed, hemp, flax, and walnut oils for use in dressings and drizzles instead. Olive and avocado oil are liquid fats too, but contain a much higher percentage of monounsaturated fats, giving them a little more stability at warmer temperatures. They're still not ideal for high-temperature cooking, but OK for light frying – softening onions and garlic, that sort of thing.

CHAPTER 4

Hydration

How many of us can say we consistently drink at least a litre and a half of plain water every day? I manage it most days, but not every day. And I can tell when I haven't.

Even a small drop in hydration levels can have a huge impact on energy, concentration, and muscle function. Headaches, fatigue, aching muscles, constipation, fluid retention (yes, if you don't drink enough, your body will hang on to what it can!), brain fog – all of these can be linked to poor hydration. Which is why drinking 1.5-2l of plain filtered (if possible) water every day is one of the cheapest and easiest positive steps you can take for your health.

Herbal infusions can count towards your total daily fluid intake and can be helpful for managing symptoms, however the bulk of your fluids ideally needs to be plain water as this is the easiest fluid for your body to digest, absorb, and use.

If you're deeply attached to your teapot or cafetière, start keeping track of how much you drink and at what time of day. We each have a unique sensitivity to caffeine, partly regulated by genetically influenced detoxification pathways in the liver, and this can alter over time. You may have been able to drink 10 coffees a day in your early 20s and still feel fine, but by your mid-40s, after a few years of stress have altered your detoxification genes, it can be a whole other story.

Caffeine is a major trigger for hot flushes, anxiety, insomnia, and mood swings. If these are some of your main symptoms, think about weaning yourself off caffeine completely – it can make a remarkable difference.

If you really can't face life without tea or coffee, switching to decaffeinated versions is a helpful first step. Opt for organic versions where possible as they don't use methylene chloride (an industrial solvent found in paint stripper and paint thinner) in the decaffeination process.

But don't stop there! Decaffeinated tea and coffee still contain low levels of caffeine which can be enough to trigger symptoms. Gradually reduce the decaff and switch to being completely caffeine free.

Here's what to drink instead …

Healthy Hydration

- Still filtered water
- Still filtered water gently flavoured with fruit slices and herbs:
    - Orange + cucumber + mint leaves
    - Lemon + lemon balm
    - Pomegranate + mint
    - Raspberries + kiwi
- Herbal infusions
    - Chamomile: soothing, calming, anti-inflammatory, antispasmodic.
    - Fennel: good for relieving trapped wind.
    - Redbush or Rooibos tea: naturally high in antioxidants whilst being caffeine free and extremely low in tannins, this is a great alternative to regular black tea.
    - Ginger: warming, anti-inflammatory, may help ease nausea.
    - Liquorice: naturally sweet, this is a perfect after dinner drink if you like to round off the meal with a sweet taste.
    - Peppermint: cooling and wind-relieving. Don't use this if you get acid reflux or heartburn.
    - Valerian: a pungent herb often combined with gentler flavours like lavender and lemon balm to help aid sleep.

- Sage: easy to grow in a garden or window box, sage has a history of traditional use for regulating body temperature and managing hot flushes.

- Lemon balm: another easy-to-grow herb, lemon balm has a delicious light flavour and combines well with fresh lemon. Drink as a warm infusion or add a few leaves to a glass of cool water. The herb has gentle soothing actions on the nervous system helping manage anxiety and tension, restlessness, mild depression, and digestive problems triggered by anxiety such as indigestion and bloating [8].

Keep a glass or stainless-steel bottle in your bag or on your work desk so you can stay hydrated throughout the day. It is far better to sip regularly than gulp down a pint in one go.

If you get so wrapped up in your day you forget to drink, download, and use, one of the water reminder apps for smartphones. You can set hourly reminders and track how much you've drunk each day – perfect for perimenopausal forgetfulness!

CHAPTER 5

Toxins & Detoxification

Hopefully, by this point you're well on your way to enjoying steadier energy levels and mood balance thanks to better blood sugar management and hydration.

Now we're going to look at the issue of toxic oestrogens – aka **xenoestrogens** – and hormone detoxification. It's important to support our detox pathways to make sure we get rid of old hormones rather than having them recycle around the body.

The term 'detox' has become synonymous with quick-fix weight loss plans and strict juicing regimes designed to purge all impurities. You may be relieved to know that's not what this chapter is about. The sort of detoxification we're talking about here is the daily processes happening in our **liver and bowels** – how we process hormones and get rid of them through poo and pee!

After oestrogen and other hormones have done their work, they end up in the liver. Here they are processed via two pathways, conveniently called Phase 1 and Phase 2.

- **Phase 1** involves getting the hormones ready to be bound up with other substances. This phase requires many different B-vitamins and is modulated in part by plant compounds found in cruciferous vegetables (broccoli, kale, cauliflower, rocket), turmeric, and berries [9].

- **Phase 2** is where the hormones are bound up or 'conjugated' to other substances ready to be eliminated from the body via poo or pee. This stage uses up lots of B-vitamins, vitamin C, magnesium, antioxidants, amino acids, and the sulphur compounds found in cruciferous vegetables and eggs, onions, and garlic.

Other toxins are being processed at the same time as hormones; for example, alcohol, medications, pesticide residues from foods, and chemicals from processed foods; all of these need to flow through the detoxification pathways. Detoxification is a constant process, and the liver is one of the most hard-working organs in the body.

At the end of Phase 2, the conjugated hormones are transported to the bowel in the bile flow. Other substances that are water-soluble are excreted via the kidneys and urine instead.

Healthy poo

This final stage of detoxification is critical. It's poo. Now the old hormones have reached the bowel, they need to be taken out of the body via bowel movements. If there is any delay here due to sluggish bowels and constipation, certain intestinal bacteria can 'de-conjugate' the hormones and send them back into circulation to the liver, thereby adding to hormonal imbalance.

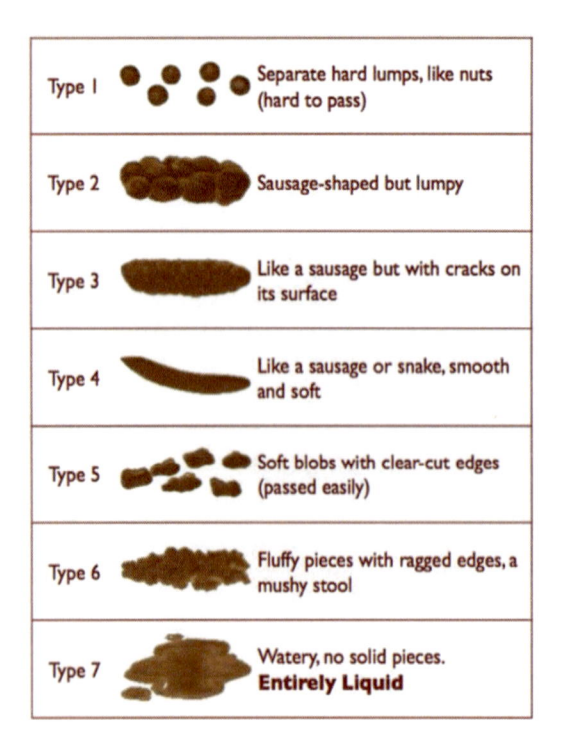

Type 1		Separate hard lumps, like nuts (hard to pass)
Type 2		Sausage-shaped but lumpy
Type 3		Like a sausage but with cracks on its surface
Type 4		Like a sausage or snake, smooth and soft
Type 5		Soft blobs with clear-cut edges (passed easily)
Type 6		Fluffy pieces with ragged edges, a mushy stool
Type 7		Watery, no solid pieces. **Entirely Liquid**

Having a healthy poo 1-3 times per day is an essential part of healthy hormone balance. And it does wonders for skin health, energy levels, bloating – pretty much every part of health is influenced by how well we poo!

Imagine never emptying the bins in your house. Think of the smell, the overflowing mess, how difficult it would be to move around your home. That's what happens inside your body when the bowels aren't working well: the waste builds up and causes a host of problems.

A **healthy poo** is sausage-shaped, dark brown in colour, easy to pass, and easy to flush away – a type 3 or 4 on the Bristol Stool Scale over there on the left.

You should feel comfortably empty afterwards; satisfied that you've passed everything.

One of the best ways to support comfortable digestion and bowel movements is to **eat mindfully**. This has already been mentioned in Chapter 3, so for a quick recap, mindful eating involves sitting down to eat, taking a few slow deep breaths to help flip your nervous system into rest-and-digest mode, and chewing each mouthful thoroughly until the food is all mushy and squishy.

These simple steps can go a long way towards alleviating bloating, excess wind, indigestion, and constipation. Remember, only your mouth has teeth: if you send big lumps of food down to your stomach, they're going to cause problems! Partially digested food is an absolute treat for some of the less-friendly bacteria living in the gut microbiota. They feed on it, producing foul smelling wind that can lead to pain, bloating, and the sort of farts that drive a dog to leave the room. So, for all our sakes, chew your food.

Comfortable bowel movements

If you're producing rabbit pellets (type 1), or hard uncomfortable logs (type 2), try these tips to make poo smoother and easier to pass:

- **Increase soluble fibre**: good sources are oats, apples, vegetables, chia seeds, and ground flaxseed. **Overnight Oats** is a great way of getting more gentle fibre into your system: mix three tablespoons of oats with one tablespoon of ground flaxseeds or chia seeds, cover with water, dairy-free/regular milk or yoghurt, and let it soak overnight. In the morning add stewed or grated apple, a handful of nuts, and fresh berries. Eat cold or gently warmed, whatever you prefer.

- **Eat hydrating foods**: vegetable soups, vegetable-based casseroles, and wholegrains and pulses that have been pre-soaked and cooked thoroughly all bring fluid and gentle fibre into the digestive system.

- **Increase water intake** – see Chapter 4 for tips on this.

- **Avoid snacking and stick to three main meals a day as much as possible.** Snacking and grazing mean your digestive system is constantly at work. There's a special wave of muscle contraction called the Migrating Motor Complex (MMC) that sweeps through your gut around 90 minutes after you've finished eating a meal. This muscle contraction pushes food and wastes along the digestive tract and helps prevent microbes and bacteria from travelling from the large intestine back up into the small intestine. Snacking and grazing interrupt this process as the MMC never gets chance to get going.

- **Give your digestive system a rest with a 12-hour overnight fast.** This is much easier than it sounds! Simply make sure you eat your three main meals and any snacks within an 12-hour window. For example, if breakfast is at 7.30am, make sure you've finished your final meal of the day by 7.30pm and forego any evening snacks – water and herbal teas are allowed. This 12-hour overnight rest period gives the cells lining your digestive tract and your microbiota (the millions of bacteria and microbes living in the gut) a chance to perform vital cellular 'housekeeping' duties without the need to process food at the same time.

- See the section on **Probiotic supplements** in Chapter 6.

If your stools are the opposite (too loose and too frequent), try the steps above but you may also need to see your GP to test for any underlying infections.

Food intolerances can contribute to both constipation and diarrhoea; wheat is a common culprit, as are dairy, egg, gluten, and soy. Identifying and managing food intolerances can be a complex process; keeping a detailed food diary for 2-3 weeks may help you identify any obvious triggers, but if there doesn't seem to be a clear pattern, get help from a registered nutritional therapist who can guide you further – see Chapter 12 for how to find a practitioner.

Please note: **if you have any sudden change in bowel habits or notice blood in your stools or on the toilet paper, see your GP for further investigations.** Our poo reveals so much about the state of our health and must not be ignored.

Xenoestrogens – how toxic oestrogens are adding to the problem

Xenoestrogens are toxic oestrogen-like substances found in bodycare products, cosmetics, perfumes, plastics, drugs, household cleaning products, non-stick coatings on pans, fire retardants, agricultural chemicals – even our water supply. These modern chemicals are flooding into our bodies and in no way have we evolved to deal with them.

These compounds mimic the effects of oestrogen – but not in a good way. Whilst they may be *structurally* similar to oestrogen, and able to latch onto oestrogen receptors, they have toxic effects. By mimicking natural oestrogen, they wreak havoc on the delicate interplay of hormones and contribute to oestrogen-dominance symptoms – which, as we mentioned in Chapter 1, can be what's happening in the early stages of perimenopause. They are also difficult to detoxify in the liver and can interfere with Phase 1 and Phase 2.

Xenoestrogens are found in tiny amounts in products, but it's the accumulative and synergistic effects of these chemicals that is most concerning. Being exposed to multiple different chemicals, many of which have not been safety tested in combination, causes a cocktail effect within our bodies and a gradual accumulation of hormone disruptors. **Consider how many products you have been exposed to already today:** scented shower gel, shampoo, perfume, body lotion, make-up, deodorant, plastic food wrapping, pesticide residues on foods, cleaning sprays, air fresheners, the non-stick coating on the pan you used to make an omelette … the list goes on.

Each trace amount of xenoestrogen accumulates in your body (mostly in fat tissue), influencing the fine balance of natural hormones at play. This vast array of toxic oestrogens is now widely considered to be a major factor in many hormonally linked conditions including autoimmune conditions and oestrogen-dependant cancers [10].

It's virtually impossible to avoid xenoestrogens because they are so ubiquitous in modern life, but we can take steps to minimise our exposure to them.

Minimising exposure to xenoestrogens

- **Switch to natural/food-based household cleaning products**. Watch out for words like 'natural' and 'green' on the labels as these can be meaningless marketing ploys used to disguise the fact that a product still contains harmful chemicals. Always read the ingredients to see what's really in the product and opt for reputable environmentally friendly brands. If you have time and enjoy concocting potions, make your own products with lemon juice, vinegar, baking soda, and essential oils – see Chapter 12 for further resources and brand suggestions.

- Swap to **chemical-free bodycare products**, make-up, and perfumes.

- Swap pesticide-sprayed cotton **tampons and sanitary towels** for organic versions or sustainable options like Mooncup, sea sponges, and reusable cloth towels.

- Where possible buy **organic produce**. This isn't always easy, accessible, or affordable, so just do what you can manage. With fruits and vegetables, a good rule of thumb is that if the food has a thick skin or peel that needs to be discarded before eating then you can get away with buying non-organic as most of the pesticide residues will be stuck in the peel. On the other hand, tiny cereal grains like rice and oats have a greater surface area for agrichemicals to stick to, so opt for organic if you can.

- The Environmental Working Group in the USA produces a 'Dirty Dozen & Clean Fifteen' list each year of the top 12 foods with the most chemical residues and the top 15 that are safe to buy as non-organic versions. It is based on produce available in the USA but is still a useful guide for other countries (see Chapter 12 – Other Therapies & Resources for details of where to find the guide).

- Don't use plastic tubs for storing foods or for microwaving; opt for **glass or ceramic containers** instead. Leftover mayonnaise and coconut oil jars are great for storing leftovers in the fridge and freezer.

- **Replace plastic water bottles** with stainless steel or glass versions.

- **Avoid non-stick pans and cookware**; opt for cast-iron, stainless steel, ceramic, or glass.

- Ditch cling film and use **beeswax wraps** instead for wrapping cheese and solid leftovers.

Some of these changes call for quite big lifestyle changes. Please don't feel alarmed or overwhelmed though, any step you take to reduce your exposure to xenoestrogens is a step in the right direction and your body will thank you for it. Just keep making gradual shifts and stick with it. In just six months you'll have significantly lowered the levels of xenoestrogens in your life.

CHAPTER 6

Essential Nutrients

All vitamins and minerals are essential to our health and well-being, but during perimenopause and menopause there are a few that need a little extra attention.

Sometimes it's difficult to get enough of the vitamins and minerals we need from foods alone. Nutrient levels in foods are not what they used to be a hundred years ago because the way we grow and store foods has changed. Intensive farming methods have depleted nutrient levels in the soil, while long transportation and storage periods mean nutrients can start to degrade before the food even reaches the stores. Because of these factors, it can be helpful to consider nutritional supplements when your body needs more than you can give it from foods alone.

Supplements are not intended to replace foods; they are designed to supplement your diet and provide a bit of back-up in times of high demand. For example, you might need extra iron because of very heavy periods or be struggling with calcium intake whilst adjusting to a dairy-free diet. If you know your diet isn't as good as it could be, you might think about taking a good quality multivitamin and mineral while you start making improvements.

The number of supplements out there is baffling and there are huge variations in price, quality, and effectiveness. No matter what the price label says, the costliest supplement is always going to be the one that doesn't work.

Here we have a handy table showing which nutrients may be needed in greater amounts during perimenopause and menopause, and the foods that supply them.

The second table shows what to look for when choosing a suitable supplement. Don't be sucked in by what's on offer on Amazon; ask for guidance at your local independent health store where the staff are trained in supplement advice and can check for any interactions between supplements and medications. You may end up paying a little more than online but at least you'll know exactly what you're taking and won't be sold some dodgy imported capsules filled with chalk powder (yes, this is used in cheap calcium supplements!).

NUTRIENT	FOOD SOURCES
ENERGY, MOOD BALANCE, HANDLING STRESS These nutrients support mental well-being and energy production	
Protein Think of protein as an all-important building block for energy and mood balance	Turkey, salmon, cottage cheese, peanuts, pumpkin seeds, sesame seeds, eggs, lentils, beef, lamb, and soy all supply tryptophan, an amino acid needed to make serotonin which helps balance mood and, in turn, converts to melatonin, a sleep hormone
Magnesium - known as the 'anti-stress mineral' because of its beneficial effects on the nervous system	Dark green leafy veg, nuts, seeds (especially pumpkin), quinoa, brown rice, avocado, dark chocolate (70%+), cacao
Vitamin B1	Pork, organ meats, salmon, tuna, seeds, peas, beans, tofu, brown rice, asparagus
Vitamin B2	Red meat, tofu, salmon, mushrooms, dairy, egg, spinach, almonds, avocado
Vitamin B3	Tuna, chicken, red meat, salmon, mushrooms, brown rice, peas, sweet potato
Vitamin B5	Shiitake mushrooms, poultry, salmon, avocado, sweet potato, tuna, egg yolk, sunflower seeds, dairy, lentils
Vitamin B6	Poultry, tuna, salmon, lentils, banana, sweet potato, spinach, peas, pistachio nuts, sunflower seeds
Folate	Leafy greens (the name folate is from the Latin for 'foliage'), lentils, beans

NUTRIENT	FOOD SOURCES
Vitamin B12	Red meat, poultry, dairy, egg, fish, fortified yeast flakes
Vitamin C	Broccoli, citrus fruit, cauliflower, kiwi, berries, peas, parsley, peppers, tomato, white potato
Iron	Red meat, poultry & shellfish for heme iron (animal source) Lentils, beans, dark-green veg, dried apricots, prunes & peaches; quinoa, pumpkin & sesame seeds, dark chocolate (70%+) for non-heme iron (plant-based)
Zinc	Poultry, red meat, shellfish, pumpkin, sunflower & hemp seeds; pecans, cashews, lentils, tofu
Omega-3 (ALA, EPA, DHA) *	EPA & DHA – Oily fish (salmon, sardines, pilchards, trout, mackerel, anchovy, herring) ALA – Ground flax & hemp seeds, flax oil, hemp oil, & walnuts

* There are two types of omega-3 oils:

ALA (alpha-linolenic acid) = the 'parent' fat, found in plant foods. This can be converted into EPA and DHA but a lot of it is lost during this process.

EPA & DHA (eicosapentaenoic acid & docosahexaenoic acid) = the 'ready-to-use' omega-3 fats needed for brain, heart, skin, and hormonal health.

BONE HEALTH	
Calcium	Full-fat dairy products (the fat provides vitamin D to aid calcium absorption); tinned fish with their small soft bones (sardines, pilchards, mackerel, salmon); Brazil nuts, almonds, sesame seeds, dried figs, broccoli, kale, spinach, okra
Vitamin D3	Oily fish, eggs, butter, milk
	Foods do not provide enough vitamin D for optimal health. Instead, we need regular sunlight exposure which is difficult in many parts of the world, including the UK. Supplementation is advisable, and essential between October and April.
	Daily supplementation all-year-round may be necessary if you have darker skin or do not expose your skin to sunlight or are housebound.
Vitamins K1 and K2	Leafy green vegetables provide vitamin K1 which can be converted to K2 in the gut.
	Certain fermented foods provide vitamin K2 (natto, butter and cheese made with milk from grass-fed cows) as does dark chicken meat and egg yolk.
Vitamin E	Sunflower seeds, almonds, olive oil, avocado, leafy green veg, wheatgerm and wheatgerm oil, trout, egg yolk
+ magnesium + zinc + vitamin C	

MANAGING INFLAMMATION
These nutrients may be helpful if you are managing any kind of inflammatory condition, particularly if it affects your joints or skin (including the vaginal lining)

Vitamin A/beta carotene	Vitamin A – liver, butter, egg yolk, dairy products
	Beta carotene (can be converted to vitamin A in the body) – red and orange veg (sweet potato, butternut squash, peppers, carrots), dried apricots, leafy green veg, peas

+ omega-3 + vitamin C + vitamin E + zinc + vitamin D3

HAIR, SKIN & NAIL HEALTH

Vitamin A/beta carotene + vitamins B1, B2, B3 + zinc + vitamin E + omega-3 + omega-7 (see supplement chart)

HOT FLUSHES

Sage (see supplement chart) + vitamin E + magnesium & the B vitamins to support the nervous system if stress is a major trigger

HEART HEALTH

Omega-3 + vitamin E + vitamin D3 + magnesium + vitamin K + vitamin B12 + folate

TABLE 2 – SUPPLEMENTS

If you are taking any medications, have a pre-existing health condition, or take other supplements of any kind, please check with a health-store advisor or a registered nutrition practitioner before using any nutritional supplements.

Vitamin D	The most usable form is D3 (cholecalciferol) which is usually derived from lanolin from sheep's wool or fish-liver oil.
	It is available in spray, capsule, tablet, or liquid form. Don't worry, there is no residual taste of sheep's wool or fish – most spray forms include peppermint oil and taste delicious!
	Vegan supplements contain either D2 from mushrooms, or D3 derived from lichen.
	What to look for
	Vitamin D can be toxic at blood levels of over 200nmol/l. As a broad guide, most adults in the UK can safely take 400–1000iu per day between October and April. However, it is a good idea to test your levels first before supplementing.
Calcium	If you have osteopenia, osteoporosis or are struggling to eat enough calcium-rich foods you may want to consider a calcium supplement.
	Calcium always needs its teammates: magnesium, vitamin D, zinc, vitamin K, boron, and manganese. For this reason, bone support formulations are particularly helpful.
	What to look for
	Like all minerals, calcium needs to be supplemented in a bioavailable form to make sure it is absorbed and used properly. Calcium citrate is an excellent choice. Avoid calcium carbonate (aka chalk) as it is poorly absorbed.
	Calcium supplements + levothyroxine (thyroid medication) – do not take these pills at the same time; leave at least two hours between them.
	Vitamin K may interfere with anticoagulant medication.

Vitamin E	Studies on vitamin E and hot flushes are limited but do show promising results[11]. A typical dosage is 400iu of alpha-tocopherol (a type of vitamin E). *Caution* Vitamin E interacts with several medications, mostly blood thinners and anticoagulants. Seek professional advice before supplementing.
Iron	Prescription iron pills are notorious for causing an upset stomach, constipation, and diarrhoea. Just what you need on top of everything else! *What to look for* Highly bioavailable and non-constipating iron bisglycinate, or food-state forms like 'Floradix'. *Caution* Iron supplements + levothyroxine (thyroid medication) – do not take these pills at the same time; leave at least two hours between them.
Omega-7	The essential fatty acid omega-7 is highly concentrated in sea buckthorn. This isn't a commonly used food item, but you can purchase capsules of the oily extract which provide high levels of omega-7. A brand leader for omega-7 is Pharma Nord which has carried out extensive research into the oil and its benefits for skin dryness, including vaginal dryness.
Probiotics	We each carry a unique blend of beneficial microbes in our digestive tract, bowel, and vagina, which can be upset by stress, illness, and medications. Taking a probiotic supplement can be useful if you: - have irritable bowel syndrome - are taking or have recently taken antibiotics - experience regular bouts of constipation or diarrhoea - experience regular urinary tract infections - experience excess bloating and wind - are experiencing prolonged stress.

There are thousands of probiotic supplements available, of varying quality and dosage. As with all supplements, it's best to get advice from a health-store advisor or registered nutrition practitioner before purchasing. Some of the good quality brands I've used myself or with clients include:

- Bio-Kult
- OptiBac
- Udo's Choice
- BioCare
- Solgar
- Nutrigold

What to look for

Most probiotic products now contain at least one billion organisms per capsule. Make sure your chosen supplement guarantees the activity of at least one billion *at the time of dosage*, and not just at the time of manufacture. There's often a big difference between how many active bacteria are present when the supplement is made and how many will be active when the product is taken.

Many brands patent particular species of bacteria that have been researched and proven to benefit certain health conditions.

Caution

You may experience a few days of wind and/or bloating when starting a course of probiotics. This is quite normal and is a sign that your gut bacteria are adjusting to the newcomers. If it is uncomfortable, reduce the dosage for a few days and then gradually increase it again.

Histamine intolerance: some probiotic species are thought to potentiate the release of histamine, though this doesn't happen to everyone who takes them. See a registered nutrition practitioner for advice if you are already dealing with excess histamine.

Some products include **prebiotics** alongside the probiotic bacteria. Prebiotics are forms of fibre that feed the bacteria, helping them to establish and thrive. If your diet includes plenty of fibre from vegetables, nuts, seeds, oats, pulses, beans, and fruits such as apples and bananas, then you may not need a supplement with prebiotics.

A commonly used prebiotic is FOS (fructooligosaccharides). It can occasionally aggravate wind and bloating; if this happens to you, try switching to an FOS-free supplement.

HERBAL REMEDIES FOR PERIMENOPAUSE

These are some of the commonly used and well-renowned herbs for perimenopausal symptoms. As with all supplements, quality is key: a cheap capsule made with the offcuts of a plant will be far less effective than an organically grown whole-herb tincture from a medical herbalist, for example.

It is important not to self-medicate with herbs owing to the risk of contraindications and interactions with other supplements or medications. For advice on over-the-counter supplements, see a trained health-store advisor, or for an herbal prescription tailored to your needs, see a registered medical herbalist.

Overview of uses

Sage	Sage: helps regulate body temperature; useful for hot flushes.
Red clover	Red clover: rich source of phytoestrogen compounds, supports hormone balance and may ease vaginal dryness and protect bones (see Chapter 7 – Phytoestrogens).
Shatavari	Shatavari: an ancient Ayurvedic herb used to balance female hormones
Black cohosh	Black cohosh: another source of oestrogen-like compounds, thought to act in a similar way to SERM (selective estrogen receptor modulator) drugs.
St. John's wort	St. John's wort: supports neurotransmitter balance in the brain, useful for mild to moderate depression.
Siberian ginseng Rhodiola Ashwagandha	Siberian ginseng, rhodiola, and ashwagandha: these are classed as 'adaptogenic' herbs that help the body adapt and cope with different physical, mental, and emotional stressors.

CHAPTER 7

Phytoestrogen Foods

Sitting alongside these essential vitamins and minerals are different types of plant-based compounds that have beneficial effects on our health. One of the most important types of compound for menopausers is **phytoestrogens**: naturally occurring substances found in fruits, vegetables, and grains, that have a similar effect to human oestrogen. They are hundreds and hundreds of times weaker than our own oestrogen and are not a hormone replacement therapy by any means. Instead, they have a **modulating** effect on our fluctuating oestrogen levels and may help reduce hot flushes and offer protection to our bones.

Phytoestrogens work by latching onto oestrogen receptors on the surface of a cell and either:

1. block the activity of human oestrogen – this is helpful during oestrogen dominance

    OR

2. provide a very weak oestrogen-like effect to the cell – this is helpful when oestrogen levels are low.

In this way, the phytoestrogens have similar actions to SERM (selective estrogen receptor modulators) drugs [12].

The three most common types of phytoestrogen are:

- **Coumestans** found in red clover and red clover sprouts, mung bean sprouts and alfalfa sprouts. These are easy to grow on the kitchen windowsill in a glass jar covered with muslin. Remember sprouting cress seeds on wet cotton wool when you were little? It's just like that! Or you can buy the fancy seed-sprouting germinator kits from BioSnacky (see Chapter 12 – Other Therapies & Resources) and have a selection of seeds and beans sprouting simultaneously. Sprouting makes the seeds and beans easier to digest and increases the bioavailability of nutrients. All the goodness that little sprout needs to grow into a larger plant becomes available to you in these tiny sprouts!

- **Lignans** found in varying amounts in a wide range of foods. Flaxseed is by far the richest source, followed by:

Top 10 lignan-rich foods (in descending order)
1. Flaxseed
2. Sesame seed
3. Broccoli
4. Cashew nuts
5. Brussel sprouts
6. Green beans
7. White cabbage
8. Red cabbage
9. Pear
10. Green sweet pepper

(Source: Rodriguez-Garcia, et al, 2019 [13])

Ground flax (also called milled or ground linseed) is the easiest form to eat as the individual seeds are so small and slippery that it's virtually impossible to chew each one properly and gain enough nutritional benefit. You can grind your own in a decent coffee grinder or buy the pre-milled seeds in a resealable packet. Store the bag in the fridge once opened as the natural seed oils can go rancid at room temperature. Aim to include 1-2 tablespoons per day for at least one month to see if it makes a difference to your symptoms. If it helps, you can continue to enjoy it for as long as you need to.

Tasty ways to use ground flax:

- Add a dessertspoonful to a homemade smoothie alongside fruit and milk.
- Mix into porridge or Overnight Oats. (See page 27 for recipe)
- Mix a tablespoonful into soup or a casserole.
- See Chapter 12 – Other Therapies & Resources for the recipes for **Menopause Cake** (yes, cake!) and dried-fruit truffle balls that include ground flaxseeds.

Fennel and fenugreek are two common herbs with phytoestrogenic properties; both can be added to meals and drunk as herbal infusions.

- **Isoflavones** found primarily in soybeans (edamame) and fermented soy products like tempeh and miso; chickpeas, aduki beans, kidney beans, and red clover. Red clover seeds can be sprouted alongside mung beans, alfalfa seeds, and chickpeas.

Soy isoflavones are the most heavily studied type of phytoestrogen and have been shown to favourably reduce hot flushes, lower LDL cholesterol, and provide a protective effect to bones [14].

However, a lot of controversy surrounds the use of soy and there are plenty of scare stories on the internet. To give this some perspective, remember that no food is entirely safe for everyone, and much of this controversial research is linked to animal studies rather than human research. In addition, the forms studied are often highly concentrated raw soy extracts, rather than traditional fermented soy products like tempeh, tofu, natto, and tamari. It is these traditional fermented soy products that offer benefits for menopausers, not the highly processed soy extracts or 'meat alternatives' like soy mince and soy burgers.

The European Food Safety Authority has looked at the issue of soy isoflavones and concluded that they do not adversely affect breast, thyroid, or uterine tissues in post-menopausal women [15].

Studies examining the effect of soy isoflavones on hot flushes are small scale but promising. For example, one study [16] compared the use of soy isoflavone supplements on women experiencing five or more hot flushes per day. This was a double-blind, randomized, placebo-controlled trial involving 40 women taking a placebo for 10 months, and 40 women using the soy isoflavone supplement. Neither group knew what they were taking, nor did the researchers, until the end of the study.

The results showed a 69.9% decrease in hot flush severity in the soy isoflavone group compared with a 33.7% reduction in the placebo group.

There were no changes in womb-lining thickness or breast tissue, and no serious adverse events related to isoflavone treatment were reported.

However, if you'd rather avoid soy, then simply include a range of other sources of isoflavones instead – there are plenty to choose from.

Isoflavones + Gut Bacteria

Not everyone responds to isoflavone-rich foods in the same way. Some find them incredibly beneficial and others see no benefit at all. It all comes down to our gut bugs. Our intestinal bacteria need to process the isoflavones and convert them into active metabolites. Because we each have a unique selection of intestinal bacteria, some menopausers are more effective at converting the isoflavones into active compounds than others, which is why some experience a benefit and others don't.

If you don't currently eat any or many of the phytoestrogen foods, introduce them gradually and keep track of your symptoms. Start with one serving of a phytoestrogen-rich food three times a week and slowly increase it to one per day. Too much too quickly may aggravate your digestion as your gut bacteria have to suddenly adapt to an increase in fibre and phytoestrogens. Better to start low and slow and increase them at your own pace.

If you're new to cooking lentils and pulses, add a strip of kombu (dried seaweed) to the pan; this can help absorb some of the gases and make them easier to digest. Dried seaweeds are available in health food stores and most larger supermarkets.

CHAPTER 8

The Essential Elements for Every Meal

Meal preparation is a wonderful opportunity to be playful and creative. Now if you're thinking "nope, I hate cooking, it's stressful and exhausting", let's reframe those thoughts …

As a practising nutritional therapist, I spent well over a decade talking about food, but I'm certainly no Master Chef. Any recipe that involves marinades or triple-cooked anything is a no. I like simple, one-pot meals that are tasty, nutritious, and have minimal washing-up.

Forget about complex recipes and cookery rules, let's strip this back and look at individual foods and how they can combine in interesting and tasty ways. Think of it like decorating: your living room needs a sofa, coffee table, and cushions, and you get to decide what colour and style they are. In much the same way, your meals need protein, complex carbohydrates, healthy fats, and plant-based compounds – and you get to choose which ones. If you consider each element individually, you can pick out five or six foods that you like, and then assemble your meal – ta dah!

For example, a breakfast of Overnight Oats made from oats, seeds, nuts, yoghurt, and fruit provides all the essential elements of protein, carbohydrates, fats, and plant-based compounds like this:

- **protein** is found in the nuts, seeds, and yoghurt
- **complex carbs** are provided mainly by the oats, though the nuts and seeds contain some complex carbs too
- **healthy fats** from the seeds and nuts

- **plant-based antioxidant compounds** come from whichever fruits you choose to add. Berries, cherries, pomegranate, and kiwi are particularly rich in antioxidant compounds and taste great as part of this dish.

Use the Essential Elements table for inspiration and see how many different and wonderful combinations you can come up with. It is only by playing and experimenting that we discover new ways of doing things. After all, who says breakfast needs to be cereal or lunch needs to be a sandwich? Mix it up and focus on the nutritional quality and delicious taste of each essential element.

Quick Guide to Portion Size

Use this diagram as a quick visual guide to check the portion proportions of veggies (plant-based compounds), complex carbohydrates, and protein sources on your plate. When it comes to fats, aim to include a small amount in each meal. This might already be as part of another food – e.g., a serving of oily fish provides protein AND healthy fats; or it might be a tablespoon of olive oil-based dressing over a salad. Not every meal will fit this template, but it's a good starting guide if you're wondering about how much of each element to include.

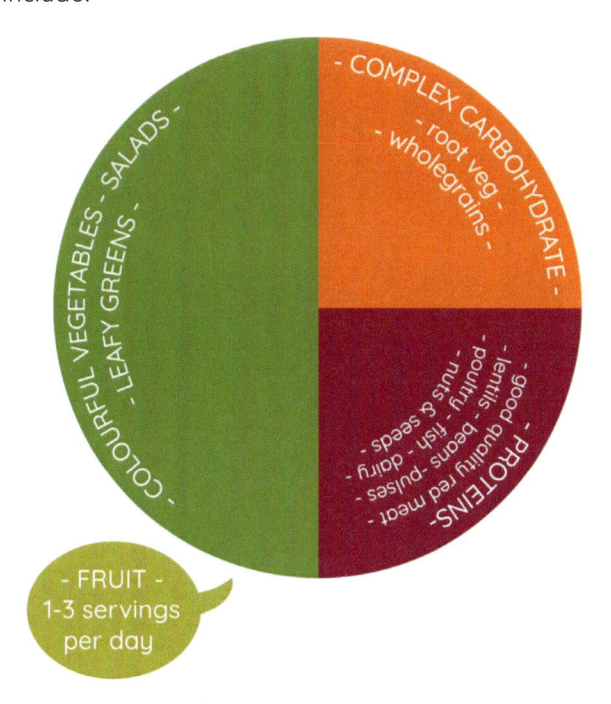

- COLOURFUL VEGETABLES - SALADS - LEAFY GREENS -
- COMPLEX CARBOHYDRATE - root veg - wholegrains -
- PROTEINS - good quality red meat - poultry - fish - dairy - lentils - beans - pulses - nuts & seeds -
- FRUIT - 1-3 servings per day

ESSENTIAL ELEMENTS FOR EACH MEAL		
ELEMENT	**FOODS**	**PORTION PROPORTIONS**
Protein	Eggs (2 eggs = a serving) Meat | Fish Full-fat dairy produce* (fat = fat-soluble vitamins) Nuts & seeds* (unsalted) Beans | Pulses | Legumes Quinoa Tofu | Tempeh	¼ of the plate
Complex carbs	Root vegetables: carrot, parsnip, beetroot, potato, sweet potato Wholegrains: e.g., brown rice, buckwheat, pot barley, oats, millet	¼ of the plate
Fats & oils	Coconut oil | butter | ghee Cold-pressed seed oils: hemp, pumpkin, flax, rapeseed Olive oil | avocado oil *Nuts, seeds, & full-fat dairy produce also contribute dietary fats	Use coconut oil, butter, or ghee for high-temperature cooking (roasting, baking) Use olive or avocado oil for light sautéing Use olive, avocado, and any of the seed oils for dressings and dips
Plant-based compounds (antioxidants, anti-inflammatory compounds, phytoestrogens)	All brightly coloured vegetables and fruits Strong colours = higher amounts of antioxidants and other protective compounds Phytoestrogens: see Chapter 7	Fill ½ the plate with colourful veggies & salad leaves Aim for 1–3 servings of fruit per day and at least 5 servings of vegetables A serving = 80g, roughly equates to 3 tablespoons of cooked veg

ELEMENT	FOODS	PORTION PROPORTIONS
Herbs & spices	Basil, coriander, chervil, chives, fennel, turmeric, rosemary, mint, lemon balm, ginger, cumin, caraway, cinnamon, lovage	Use liberally, as often as possible. Great for adding flavour, variety, and increasing diversity

CHAPTER 9

Sleep

Getting a good night's sleep feels virtually impossible when hot flushes, anxiety, and insomnia are in full flow. Lack of sleep affects every system in your body – digestion, energy levels, mood, weight balance, immunity, hormones – and, of course, feeling tired makes you crave more sleep. It is the very definition of a vicious circle.

Oestrogen receptors are found throughout the brain including in the suprachiasmatic nucleus, the tiny part of the brain responsible for setting and organising our circadian rhythms – our 24-hour internal clock that regulates sleeping, waking, eating, exercising; pretty much everything we do. Once oestrogen starts to drop, all these patterns can be affected – especially sleep.

Managing lack of sleep can be incredibly hard because it demands radical self-kindness. You absolutely must cut yourself some slack during the day. Don't overfill your schedule. Delegate tasks. Take naps if possible or sit or lie comfortably and follow a guided meditation for 20mins. These pockets of rest can give you the boost you need to make it through to bedtime.

Follow the steps for hydration in Chapter 4 and blood sugar balance in Chapter 3 as they both significantly influence sleep. Alongside those suggestions, work your way through these sleep tips. Do as many as you can and keep a note of how successful they are so that you know which ones are worth embedding into your routine.

Sleep Support

- Stick to a regular bedtime and wake-up time, including on weekends and days off. Rather than pressuring yourself to stick to an *exact* time – "It's 10.36pm, I need to be in bed in exactly four minutes!"

- set yourself a half-hour window for flexibility, e.g., bed between 10.30-11pm, getting up between 7-7.30am. Your body loves regular rhythms and by sticking to a pattern you are giving yourself the *opportunity* for sleep, even if sleep doesn't always happen.

- Avoid staring at screens for at least 1hr before bed: TV, phone, iPad, tablet – the whole lot. Screens emit blue light waves that disrupt the production of melatonin, our sleep timing hormone. Go old school and curl up with a book or magazine instead. If you do need to use a screen close to bedtime, invest in a pair of amber glasses. The coloured lenses filter out short wave blue light, reducing the impact on melatonin production.

- Aim to be in bed ready to sleep by 11pm at the latest. We get more of the slow-wave deep sleep earlier on in the night and late bedtimes (i.e., after 11pm) deprive you of it.

- Keep your bedroom cool (ideally 18°C) and dark. Fit a dimmer switch to the bedroom light to keep light levels low if you need to get up during the night. A sleep mask can be incredibly helpful during summer when the sun rises early, or if there's a street lamp outside your window.

- Wear loose cotton night clothes to allow your skin to breathe or try some of the new ranges of temperature-control nightwear that wick sweat away – see Chapter 12 for a list of suppliers.

- Swap the duvet for layers of blankets so you can adjust bed temperature more easily. If you're sharing the bed with a partner who has a vastly different body temperature, try the split weight 'Hot & Not' duvet from Nanu Sleep (see Chapter 12 for more details) or a temperature-regulating mattress protector. You may find linen sheets more comfortable and cooling than cotton or polycotton.

- Include food sources of melatonin in any afternoon snacks and your evening meal. Melatonin is one of several sleep signallers the brain produces to get us to sleep. It is the change in light in the late afternoon/evening (depending on the time of year) that tells the brain to start producing melatonin. As the sun drops, our eyes detect the lower light, and that tiny part of the brain – the suprachiasmatic nucleus – sets a cascade of signals in motion that eventually gets us to sleep.

Artificial light blocks the signal to produce melatonin (but doesn't block other parts of the cascade, which is why we still feel sleepy even when working on screens till late), as do high levels of cortisol, the stress hormone. Including food sources of melatonin is a good way of supporting levels of this sleep hormone, and whilst it won't remedy insomnia overnight, it's a helpful part of a longer-term plan.

- Foods rich in melatonin [17]:

    - pistachio nuts
    - kidney beans
    - almonds
    - fennel
    - oats
    - tart cherries (available as Montmorency cherry juice)
    - strawberries
    - salmon.

- Go for a 30min morning walk. Enjoying natural morning light even on cloudy days means your eyes are better equipped to detect the change in light at dusk and send signals to the brain to start releasing melatonin.

- Avoid caffeine (see Chapter 4 – Hydration) and opt for a mug or two of a relaxing herbal infusion: valerian, chamomile, lime blossom, and lemon balm are renowned for their calming properties and can aid sleep.

- Avoid alcohol. Having a drink in the evening can make you feel sleepy at first, but this is a false sense of security. Alcohol disrupts sleep patterns (especially the rapid eye movement phase of sleep), increases the likelihood of snoring, and can cause a drop in blood sugar – all of which prevent a good night's sleep.

- Allow at least three hours between finishing your evening meal and going to bed. Eating close to bedtime can trigger symptoms of heartburn and reflux when you lie down to sleep.

- Scatter a few drops of pure lavender oil or chamomile oil on your pillow. (NB – if you have any concerns about sensitivities to essential oils please consult a qualified aromatherapist before using them.)

- Listen to a guided meditation: a soothing voice provides a welcome distraction from anxious repeating thoughts, helping you drift off to sleep.

- Australian Bush Flower Essences or Bach Flower Remedies can be useful for dealing with emotional worries that may be contributing to sleeplessness – see Chapter 12 for more details.

- In Ayurvedic medicine, rosewater is used as a cooling remedy, particularly suited to perimenopausal hot flushes. Keep a spray bottle by the bed to spritz your face, neck, and chest as soon as a flush begins.

If all else fails and you find yourself lying awake for more than half an hour, get up, keep the lights low, and move to another room where you can read for a short while. Or knit. Or do a jigsaw. Or anything else that's calming, repetitive, and doesn't involve using a screen. After 30 minutes or so, go back to bed and try again.

Keeping a **sleep journal** for a month can be a useful way of highlighting any consistent interruptions. Make note of what time you go to bed, how well you sleep, and the time(s) you get up. You can do this with pen and notepad (any excuse to buy more notebooks!) or use one of the many sleep-tracking apps available now. Watch out for any correlations between poor sleep and stress, foods, alcohol, and your menstrual cycle.

CHAPTER 10

Movement

This one can feel particularly challenging when you have no energy, but bear with me here. Enjoying different forms of movement each day is vital for our mental, physical, and emotional well-being, especially so during perimenopause when we are experiencing so much upheaval.

A sedentary lifestyle is literally a killer. Lack of regular movement and exercise leads to loss of muscle tone, weight gain, sluggish circulation, and an increased risk of chronic diseases like heart disease [18] and osteoporosis. We need to get our blood pumping, lymph flowing, and limbs moving every single day - even when we're tired - because movement helps stimulate energy, circulation, and the release of uplifting mood chemicals.

Maintaining bone strength is crucial both during and after menopause. Sitting for long periods of time does nothing to help our bones. Bone strength relies on bone-building cells being stimulated by impact movement; when your foot hits the floor it sends signals to bone cells instructing them to build bone tissue to keep your skeleton strong. We need to keep moving if we want our bones to last; brisk walking, jogging, tennis, dancing - these are all good options for supporting bone health and reducing the risk of osteoporosis.

Maintaining healthy muscle is just as important. We start to lose muscle mass after menopause because of the drop in oestrogen and testosterone, and this has consequences for weight balance and overall strength. Muscle tissue is more metabolically active than fat and influences our basal metabolic rate, i.e., the number of calories we burn each day just by existing. If we can build and maintain our muscle tissue, we burn more calories even when we're sitting watching Netflix.

Resistance exercises are key for muscle maintenance. These include:

- Using wrist and/or ankle weights when out walking.
- Using strength bands.
- Kettlebell training.
- Body weight exercises like plank, squats, or press-ups. If press-ups sound daunting, try doing them standing up and leaning against a wall, or doing them with your knees on the floor rather than having your legs outstretched.
- Swimming or Aquafit classes.

One muscle that gets overlooked until it starts to weaken is the **pelvic floor** – the sling-shaped muscle holding all the pelvic cavity organs in place. It can become weakened by pregnancy, childbirth, menopause, and straining caused by chronic constipation, leading to bladder and/or bowel incontinence. If you are concerned about your pelvic floor talk to your GP practice nurse or see a specialist physiotherapist trained in pelvic floor health to discuss specific exercises – see Chapter 12 for details of specialist help.

Yoga is wonderful for strength, flexibility, and balance – both physically and mentally. A yoga session is a true workout for body and mind! Hatha- and Scaravelli-style classes are good for beginners, while Ashtanga is a little more advanced. It's a good idea to attend a class or have a 1-1 session with a yoga teacher before starting to practice at home to make sure you're holding the postures correctly and not overdoing any stretches. The last thing you want is a yoga-induced injury messing up your exercise plans.

The most important point is to **enjoy movement** every day – outdoors preferably, to get the benefit of natural light and fresh air, even in cold weather! Mix up your options. Do activities with a friend for extra accountability and a few laughs. Find the thing that makes you smile and look forward to doing it again.

Regularity and consistency are key when it comes to establishing a **new movement habit**. To help this new habit take hold, pick a couple of time slots in the week when you can do longer bouts, get them in your diary, then look at fitting in mini pockets of movement around these. For example:

- 60min yoga class on Tuesday
- 30 minutes swimming on Saturday morning
- intersperse 20min walks in your lunch hour and 10min bursts of dancing in the kitchen while making tea every day.

And remember, whatever gets you moving is keeping you well.

CHAPTER 11

Emotional Support

Menopause is called 'the change' for lots of reasons, not just because our child-bearing days are over. It can be a time of huge emotional upheaval caused only in part by the crazy dancing hormones. Perimenopause and menopause often coincide with changes in career, children leaving home, or parents and older relatives becoming frail or unwell and in need of care. Many menopausers feel 'sandwiched' between the demands of their jobs, offspring, and parents: pulled in competing directions with little time to focus on their own needs.

During perimenopause and after menopause our emotional perspective can change.

Our priorities can change.

How we feel about our bodies can change.

You might feel waves of joy and a newfound zest for life now that periods are ending. Or you may experience sadness, regret, loneliness, and unexpected bouts of crying.

You might feel distanced from your partner. Or closer than ever before.

You might be struggling with low libido. Or you might be on fire and wanting sex more than ever.

You might be exhausted all day. Or, you might be dancing round the kitchen and having an absolute blast.

It's your own emotional rollercoaster – but that doesn't mean you have to ride it alone. This is a challenging time and you're going to need resilience and a support team to get through it.

Build Your Resilience

Resilience describes our ability to adapt and cope physically, mentally, and emotionally with challenging circumstances. When we're resilient, we have the strength and stamina to cope with upheavals: they may knock us, exhaust us, and cause a few teary meltdowns, but ultimately, we can adapt, grow, and carry on.

If we think of resilience as being like the power reserves in a battery pack, it makes sense to think of ways to create, conserve and maintain this power.

Simple steps to creating and nurturing resilience

- **Accepting change as a necessary part of life**. Yes, menopause can be deeply uncomfortable – unwanted even – and we have no say over how long it will last. However, fighting it just makes life harder. Once we accept change of any kind, we can adapt and learn to flow with it, and grow as a result. Mindfulness and meditation practices can be enormously helpful for learning about acceptance (see below).

- Developing **self-awareness** through listening to your body and paying attention to emotional, physical, and spiritual needs.

- **Setting aside time each day to focus on YOU**. This could be enjoying a long lazy bath, going to a yoga class, reading, taking a walk in the park, or sitting and listening to your favourite tunes. You might book a regular session with a reflexologist, masseur, or Reiki practitioner. The important thing is that this time is **protected** – it's yours and everyone else knows not to interrupt you.

- **Practising mindfulness**: the art of being in this moment and recognising this is all there is. It's a hugely liberating and empowering practice, brilliant for managing anxiety and mood swings. There are many apps and books to help with this; see Chapter 12 for more details.

- **Practising meditation**: there are lots of forms of meditation, none of which require you to empty your mind and think of nothing because that's impossible – if we had empty minds, we'd be dead! There are walking meditations, guided meditations, seated meditations, meditations to manage anxiety, meditations for gratitude – endless options! And again, there are books, apps, classes, and videos to help you learn. This is a fantastic practice for building resilience.

- **Journaling**: getting your thoughts and feelings out onto paper helps you maintain perspective and is wonderfully cathartic. Write what you like; these notes are for your eyes only. If you're really concerned about someone else reading your words, use loose-leaf paper and tear it up afterwards.

- Work on **sleep habits** (see Chapter 9).

Select your support team

Look around you. Who else do you know who may be a menopauser?

If you're working your way through this book with a friend, can you create time for talking and tackling emotional concerns?

Can you chat to an older friend or relative who remembers what it's like to go through this process?

Build your own support team by finding people who listen well; partner, friends, family, co-workers, online support groups, counselling services – whoever you feel comfortable chatting with. They might have direct experience of menopause or maybe they don't have a clue but happen to be a wonderful, empathic listener. You may well find others who are struggling and glad of the chance to talk and find support too. Only by talking openly about menopause can we break down the stigma that surrounds it.

See the next chapter for further details about counselling services and menopause support groups.

CHAPTER 12

Other Therapies & Resources

Here you will find a selection of resources to support you on your path through perimenopause and beyond. The brands and products mentioned below are included because I have either used them myself, have had them recommended to me by people I know and trust, or am impressed by their good reputation. There are no affiliate links here, no paid-for product placements.

Find a Nutrition Practitioner

Currently, 'nutritional therapist' is not a protected working title in the UK, which means anyone can call themselves one. There's a wide variety of training courses and qualifications available ranging from online certificates to three-year master's degrees. Whoever you contact, be sure to ask about their training, qualifications, and ongoing professional development. You may be able to find this information on their website if they have one.

The leading professional bodies for nutrition practitioners are:

British Association for Nutrition & Lifestyle Medicine (BANT): go to www.bant.org.uk and click on 'Find a Practitioner'. BANT now requires all new registrants to hold a nutrition qualification at degree level or above, and many members are qualified to master's level.

Federation of Nutritional Therapy Practitioners – www.fntp.org.uk

Naturopathic Nutrition Association – www.nna-uk.com

Counselling

British Association for Counselling and Psychotherapy – www.bacp.co.uk

BACP is listed on the Stonewall directory of Diversity Champions, organisations that are recognised as being aware of the specific needs of LGBTQ service users.

Counselling Directory – www.counselling-directory.org.uk

Also search for counselling services in your local area. There are hundreds of groups offering local 1-1 support.

Online & face-to-face menopause support & resources

Gen M www.gen-m.com

Founded by Sam Simister and Heather Jackson, Gen M curates news, research, and resources for everyone experiencing menopause. Sam and Heather surveyed 2000 UK women aged 35-60 to find out what they knew about menopause, how they felt about it, and what they needed. The results became the ground-breaking white paper 'Generation Menopause – The Invisibility Report 2020'. The paper is a wake-up call to retailers, brands, manufacturers, and employers about the needs of menopausers, as well as a rallying cry from these 'invisible' mid-life women.

Menopause Cafés: started in Scotland in 2017 by Rachel Weiss, the café gatherings and are now held all over the world. Open to anyone affected by, or wanting to know more about menopause, they take place in accessible venues and provide a safe confidential space to discuss menopause and find help and support. Find out more and search for a gathering near you at www.menopausecafe.net

British Menopause Society: telephone and email support, plus newsletters and factsheets are available from www.womens-health-concern.org, the patient arm of the British Menopause Society.

Positive Pause: a website dedicated to empowering menopausers at all stages of menopause. Packed with informative blogs and videos, Positive Pause also offers menopause training for organisations: www.positivepause.co.uk

The Daisy Network at www.daisynetwork.org provides specific support for premature ovarian insufficiency (POI) and early menopause.

Menopause Matters forum is at www.menopausematters.co.uk, where you can chat, ask questions, share ideas and tips.

Online chat with others sharing their experiences of menopause is available at **Menopause ChitChat**: https://forum.menopausechitchat.com

Vaginal lubricants

'Yes' offer a wide range of lubricant products, some of which are currently available on prescription in the UK: www.yesyesyes.org

Jane Lewis discusses her personal experience of living with the painful and debilitating condition vaginal atrophy in her book *Me & My Menopausal Vagina*. Find out more at www.mymenopausalvagina.co.uk

Pelvic floor health

Search for a female health physiotherapist in your area.

The **Squeezy app** www.squeezyapp.com is an award-winning app designed by chartered physiotherapists specialising in pelvic floor health exercise programmes.

Adore Your Pelvic Floor is an online and in-person programme created by women's health & fitness professional Louise Field and supported by a specialist physiotherapist. Find out more at www.adoreyourpelvicfloor.co.uk

Mindfulness & building resilience

The mental health charity Mind has a wealth of information on managing stress and building resilience; search 'how to manage stress' and 'developing resilience' at www.mind.org.uk

There's a wide range of smartphone apps offering guided meditations and mindfulness techniques. Popular ones include:

- Let's Meditate (free to use, option available to donate)
- Headspace
- Happy Not Perfect
- Calm
- Insight Timer

Acupuncture, medical herbalism, yoga, and holistic therapies

Traditional Chinese Medicine acupuncture is an established therapy for all aspects of perimenopause and menopause, backed by research. Find a practitioner near you via the British Acupuncture Council at www.acupuncture.org.uk

Australian Bush Flower Essences: www.ausflowers.co.uk

Bach Flower Remedies: www.bachcentre.com

National Institute of Medical Herbalists: www.nimh.org.uk

Federation of Holistic Therapists: the UK's largest professional association for holistic and complementary therapists. Use their 'Find A Therapist' facility to find a therapist near you. Therapies include massage, Reiki, hypnotherapy, reflexology, aromatherapy and many more: www.fht.org.uk

Hypnotherapy: General Hypnotherapy Standards Council & General Hypnotherapy Register: www.general-hypnotherapy-register.com/

Find a **yoga** class near you with a British Wheel of Yoga practitioner at www.bwy.org.uk

Managing toxins

Homemade household cleaning products

Pinterest is full of hints and tips for making your own cleaning products, most of which are based around Castile soap, baking soda, white vinegar, and lemon juice.

The Green Parent magazine has a good round-up of ideas at: www.thegreenparent.co.uk/articles/read/make-your-own-cleaning-products

As does Friends of the Earth: www.friendsoftheearth.uk/lifestyle/homemade-cleaning-products-5-fantastic-recipes

Bodycare products

It's possible to make your own toothpaste, deodorant, moisturiser, lip balm, bath bomb, soap – pretty much any bodycare product – at home. One of my favourite tips came from a nutrition and toxins expert who swore by her own lip tint made from coconut oil and natural beetroot-derived pink food colouring! Simply search 'homemade bodycare' for ideas.

If you'd rather leave it to the professionals, there's no shortage of brands offering high quality ethical products made with 100% plant-based ingredients and no chemical nasties. A few of my favourites are:

Holistic Kitchen: www.holistickitchen.co.uk

Totally Natural Skincare: www.totallynaturalskincare.co.uk

Neal's Yard Remedies: www.nealsyardremedies.com

INIKA Organic (make-up): www.inikaorganic.com

The 'Clean Fifteen & Dirty Dozen'. Every year the Environmental Working Group in the US produces a list of the top 15 fruits and vegetables which are considered safe enough to buy non-organically, and the top 12 which are recommended to buy as organics. Some of the information is slightly different here in the UK, but the list provides a good rule-of-thumb guide. Sign up to receive the free list at www.ewg.org/foodnews/clean-fifteen.php

Fruit & vegetable box schemes

Riverford Organic Farmers and Abel and Cole are popular national organic food delivery services, and you may find local ones in your area.

Riverford Organic Farmers: www.riverford.co.uk

Abel & Cole: www.abelandcole.co.uk

Seed and bean sprouting kits: search for BioSnacky products at www.avogel.co.uk

Sleep Support: bed linen & nightwear to keep you cool and comfortable
Nanu Sleep: the 'Hot&Not' split-weight duvet: www.nanusleep.co.uk

DermaTherapy: bedding designed to reduce dampness and clamminess and aid restful sleep: www.dermatherapybedding.co.uk

Become: a range of clothing designed for menopausal women including the Anti-Flush camisole and leggings designed to wick sweat away, cool the skin, minimise odour, and release heat back onto the skin during the post-flush cold chill. Available at www.becomeclothing.com

Cucumber: a range of UK-made stylish sleep, lounge, and daywear designed to be breathable, sustainable, long-lasting and quick drying. Available at www.cucumberclothing.com

Recipes

Start the Day Smoothie

Blend:
1 small banana OR handful of strawberries/blueberries/raspberries
Generous handful of baby spinach
1 dessertspoon of nut butter (almond, cashew, hazel, or peanut)
1 tablespoon ground flaxseeds
300ml milk of your choice

Optional extras:
1 teaspoon raw cacao powder for a chocolaty hit
1 teaspoon spirulina powder for protein and antioxidants
1 tablespoon kefir (water or dairy) for a fermented foods boost

If you don't want to drink it all in one go, save the rest in a glass bottle in the fridge for up to two days. The ground flaxseeds will soak up some of the liquid if left in the fridge so you may need to add more milk depending on how thick you like your smoothie.

Lunch Box

Pick a base: 3 tablespoons of any combination of: cooked quinoa/cooked pasta (regular or gluten-free)/cooked brown rice.

Add protein: palm-sized piece of good quality cooked meat or fish/2 hard-boiled eggs/3 tablespoons cooked lentils/nuts & seeds.

Add a mixture of raw and cooked veggies in as many colours as possible.

Top with a sprinkling of nuts and seeds (if you haven't added them already), pomegranate seeds, fresh chopped herbs.

Drizzle with homemade dressing.

Homemade dressing

3 tablespoons cold-pressed oil – olive, flax, hemp, pumpkin seed, or avocado

Juice and rind of 1 lemon

1 tablespoon apple cider vinegar with the mother (the cloudy looking mass of beneficial bacteria that turns the apple juice into vinegar)

1 teaspoon wholegrain mustard (optional)

Put all the ingredients in a glass jar and shake thoroughly to mix. Store in a cool dry place for up to three days.

Autumn Glow Soup

This soup is rich in beta-carotene, a powerful antioxidant needed for immunity and skin health. It's called 'Autumn Glow' because squashes come into season then, but you can make it at any time of year.

500g carrots, peeled and diced
500g butternut squash, peeled and diced
Generous sized piece of root ginger (about the size of the end of your thumb) peeled and grated
1 large onion peeled and chopped
1 teaspoon paprika
1 teaspoon ground cumin
Ground black pepper – to taste
1-2 teaspoons ghee/coconut oil
250ml passata
1.5-2l vegetable stock
Optional: soya or cashew cream to drizzle

Melt the ghee or coconut oil in a large pan. Once warmed, add the onion and cook gently for 5 minutes. Add the spices and ginger and stir well.

Add all the vegetables and passata, stir well, and cook for 2 minutes. Add the stock, bring to the boil, then simmer until vegetables are soft.

Allow to cool, then blend till smooth.

Serve with an extra dash of black pepper and a drizzle of soya or cashew cream.

Menopause Cake – makes two loaves

200g wholemeal flour (gluten-free plain flour or buckwheat flour could be substituted for a gluten-free alternative)
100g porridge oats
100g golden flaxseeds
50g sunflower seeds
50g sesame seeds
50g flaked almonds
2 pieces chopped stem ginger
200g raisins
750ml organic soya milk or almond milk
1 tbsp malt extract
½ teaspoon each of nutmeg, cinnamon and ground ginger.

Stir all the dry ingredients together in a large mixing bowl. Add the milk and malt extract and leave to soak for 30mins. If the mixture is very stiff, add more soya or almond milk. Spoon the mixture into two lightly oiled and lined loaf tins and bake at 190°C/375°F/gas mark 5 for about 75mins or until cooked through. Turn out and leave to cool. Enjoy a slice a day. To keep the cake fresh, slice and freeze. Defrost as needed.

Dried Fruit Truffle Balls

1 cup of chopped dried fruit; dates, figs and/or apricots work well
½ cup oats and/or cashew nuts
½ tsp vanilla extract
2 tspn raw cacao powder
Desiccated coconut and ground flaxseeds for coating

Whizz all the ingredients together in a blender. Shape into small balls and coat in the coconut and flaxseeds. Truffles will keep for up to a week in your fridge.

Acknowledgments

This book is inspired by each and every menopauser I have had the pleasure of working with in my nutrition practice. Thank you all.

Thank you to my wonderful friends and family who have believed in me and provided endless support and ideas. To Tom and Owen, Mum, Dad, Jess, Rob, Louie, and Fearn. To the brilliant Barefooters – Michelle, Joe, Gayle, and Bridget – and to Jules. Without you all, my business and this book would not be possible.

Thank you to all the early readers of this book for your thoughtful, kind, and constructive feedback that helped reshape and refine each chapter. And thanks to my friends and colleagues in the nutrition and natural health industry who willingly share their knowledge and experience for the betterment of all.

Special thanks to Michelle Hughes at Michelle Hughes Design for interpreting my toddler-like sketch into the clear and colourful diagram in Chapter 8. www.michellehughesdesign.com

And thanks to you, for reading.

References

[1] Hill A. 2020. Female doctors in menopause retiring early due to sexism, says study. *The Guardian* [online]. https://www.theguardian.com/society/2020/aug/06/female-doctors-in-menopause-retiring-early-due-to-sexism-says-study?utm_term=7f23e9371b1c6bf21e8f38491f6ada15&utm_campaign=TheWeekInPatriarchy&utm_source=esp&utm_medium=Email&CMP=weekinpatriarchy_email [Accessed 18th August 2020]

[2] Newson L. 2018. Menopause and cardiovascular disease. *Post Reproductive Health* 24(1) 44–49. doi.org/10.1177/2053369117749675

[3] Ibid.

[4] Powell, Jessica (private communication).

[5] Jones L. 2019. Women get half the number of heart attack treatments as men. *British Heart Foundation* [online]. https://www.bhf.org.uk/what-we-do/news-from-the-bhf/news-archive/2019/october/women-get-half-the-number-of-heart-attack-treatments-as-men [Accessed 25/04/2020]

[6[Gersh F. 2020. An untold heartfelt story: oestrogen and cardiac health. BANT conference [online] 7 March 2020.

[7] Mosconi L. 2020. How menopause affects the brain [video online]. https://www.youtube.com/watch?v=JJZ8z_nTCZQ [Accessed 11th August 2020]

[8] Perry, N. & Perry E. 2018. *Botanical Brain Balms.* Brighton: Filbert Press.

[9] Hodges R. E. & Minich D. M. 2015. Modulation of Metabolic Detoxification Pathways Using Foods and Food-Derived Components: A Scientific Review with Clinical Application. *Journal of Nutrition and Metabolism* 760689. doi.org/10.1155/2015/760689

[10] Patel S., Homaei A., Raju A. B. & Meher B. R. 2018. Estrogen: The necessary evil for human health, and ways to tame it. *Biomedicine & Pharmacotherapy* 102, 403-411. doi: 10.1016/j.biopha.2018.03.078

[11] Ziaei S., Kazemnejad A. & Zareai M. 2007. The Effect of Vitamin E on Hot Flashes in Menopausal Women. *Gynecologic and Obstetric Investigation* 64(4), 204-207. doi.org/10.1159/000106491

[12] Ososki A. L. & Kennelly E. J. 2003. Phytoestrogens: a review of the present state of research. *Phytotherapy Research* 17(8), 845-869.

[13] Rodríguez-García C., Sánchez-Quesada C., Toledo E., Delgado-Rodríguez M. & Gaforio J. J., 2019. Naturally Lignan-Rich Foods: A Dietary Tool for Health Promotion? *Molecules* 24(5), 917. doi:10.3390/molecules24050917

[14] Arena S., Rappa C., Del Frate E., Cenci S., & Villani C. 2002. A natural alternative to menopausal hormone replacement therapy. Phytoestrogens. [Abstract only – article in Italian] *Minerva Ginecologica* 54(1), 53-7.

[15] Messina M. 2016. Soy and Health Update: Evaluation of the Clinical and Epidemiologic Literature. *Nutrients* 8(12), 754. doi: 10.3390/nu8120754

[16] Nahas E. A. P., Nahas-Neto J., Orsatti F. L., Carvalho E. P., Oliveira M. L. C. S. & Dias R. 2007. Efficacy and safety of a soy isoflavone extract in postmenopausal women: a randomized, double-blind, and placebo-controlled study [Abstract only] [online]. *Maturitas* 58(3), 249-58. Epub 2007. https://www.ncbi.nlm.nih.gov/pubmed/17913408 [Accessed 07/03/2020]. [DOI:https://doi.org/10.1016/j.maturitas.2007.08.012 gives direct link]

[17] Meng X., Li Y., Li S., Zhou Y., Gan R.-Y., Xu D.-P., Li H.-B. 2017. Dietary Sources and Bioactivities of Melatonin. *Nutrients* 9(4), 367. doi: 10.3390/nu9040367

[18] Kubota Y., Evenson K. R., Maclehose R. F., Roetker N. S., Joshu C. E., & Folsom A. R. (2017). Physical Activity and Lifetime Risk of Cardiovascular Disease and Cancer. *Medicine & Science in Sports & Exercise* 49(8), 1599-1605. https://doi.org/10.1249/MSS.0000000000001274

About the Author

Sally Duffin is a writer and registered nutritionist (MBANT) with special interests in nutrition & lifestyle support for gut, brain, and perimenopausal health. She lives in York, England, with her husband and son.

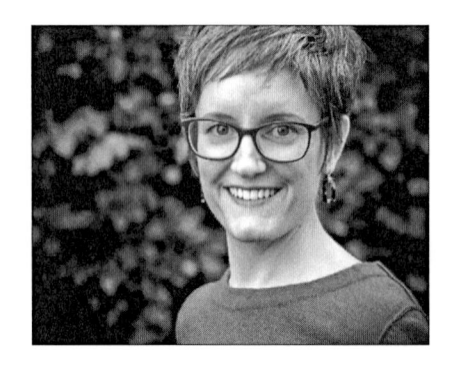

Connect with Sally on:

    Facebook - search 'Nutrition in York'

    Twitter - @nutritioninyork

    Website - www.nutritioninyork.co.uk

Please note: Sally is unable to give personalised advice via email or social media.